T0195070

MIND AND MUSCLE

CHANGE YOUR MIND, CHANGE YOUR BODY, CHANGE YOUR LIFE

SEAN YAGHOTIAN

authorHOUSE®

AuthorHouse™
1663 Liberty Drive
Bloomington, IN 47403
www.authorhouse.com
Phone: 833-262-8899

Published by AuthorHouse 03/15/2021

ISBN: 978-1-6655-1423-1 (sc)
ISBN: 978-1-6655-1424-8 (hc)
ISBN: 978-1-6655-1441-5 (e)

Library of Congress Control Number: 2021901106

CONTENTS

PREFACE

Growing up, I had a strong desire for sports and fitness, as well as topics of meditation and mindfulness. I started my active journey with running and basketball, which I was passionate about. Furthermore, I had a more in-depth desire to activate my inner dimensions through meditation, yoga, and various other practices. Through sports, I quickly learned about the relationship between the mind and body, and that motivated me to continue my research.

Throughout my life, I have tried to understand and comprehend the connection between the mind and the physical body, as well as our spiritual dimensions; these concepts have been at the core of my journey up until this day. Human anatomy is multifaceted and complex, and with all the advancements in science and technology today, we are still evolving, and the more we go forward, the more we realize there is so much more to go. Just like in space, it is infinite and boundless.

Ever since I was a teenager, I always knew there had to be more to life than the cellular level that I had experienced. I always felt it was my mission to make a difference. Although my journey has not been easy through my struggles as a human along with many trials and failures, the one thing that has kept me going is my deeper desire to be more and to understand life the way God designed it for us.

Today, through my research in various studies as well as books like *Mind and Body*, I plan on deeply exploring human anatomy both physically, psychologically, as well as spiritually. I believe if these three dimensions are not in tuned with one another, one will not be able to experience self-awareness or the essence of life. My studies are focused on finding ways to modernize this process for all people, and *Mind and Body* will guide you along the way with me.

INTRODUCTION

"For me, exercise is more than just physical –
it's therapeutic."

~Michelle Obama

Truer words have never been spoken. Fitness and exercise go beyond more than challenging the body; they challenge the mind. Also, if exercise is capable of changing your mind, mood, and attitude, then it can change your life.

Rarely, will you find an individual who devotes his life to exercising living a miserable life, and why is that? Is it more than just running a few blocks every day or visiting the gym regularly? Does it involve more than an intentional movement of body parts? Does it provide more than health and physical benefits? Yes! You'd be surprised if you knew all of distinct ways exercising could improve your body, relationship, and personality.

Are you a young person looking for motivation to work out to stay young and happy? Are you a mid-professional person working a corporate job and starting a family, not knowing how to balance both? Are you someone who wishes to build his or her personality in preparation for your present or future family or people surrounding you? Are you just seeking knowledge about how and why to exercise? Then you don't need to search any further for answers!

Almost everyone would love to exercise; we all want to have a perfect and attractive body while staying healthy. However, most people find it hard to consistently make a few miles run every morning or attend the gym every day. Several books have been written about fitness and how it helps the body; however, the therapeutic portion has been mostly left out of the benefits of exercising. What *Mind and Muscle: Change Your Mind Change Your Body Change Your Life* explains and teaches is far more than you would find on the local websites about fitness and exercise. By the time you finish reading this book, your mentality and perception about exercising will have changed.

In order to gain the most insight from this book, keep your mind open and flexible to accept new facts, ideas, and beliefs. Many people have gone down similar roads before, and they end up unchanged or undecided about who they want to be. You shouldn't end up that way; all you need is a mind that is ready to learn and progress. Strap on your headband and lace up your sneakers—it's quite a long journey, so let's get started!

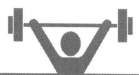

CHAPTER 1

EARLY DEVELOPMENT

"Children are not things to be molded, but are people to be unfolded."

~ Jess Lair

It seems necessary to start the journey with a little background information and education about human habits to ensure a comprehensive understanding for later discussions. The decisions we make have a way of shaping our lives in the long run.

Humans are wired to learn and adapt. Unfortunately, we don't come with a ready-made personality or way of life; we have to live by the kind of education we get from our environment during childhood. That's the major reason it is unexpected for someone who was raised in the east to think or reason exactly the way someone raised in the west would. Our childhood determines a lot about our adulthood. Basically, our family, life stages, environment, culture, conduct, diet, and all other determining factors we experience during childhood lead to our long-term habit as an adult.

Why is this early development very important? It is essential because it is connected to a lot of traits in our lives, such as our productivity, logical reasoning, sociability, cognitive skills, psychological behavior, biological performance, and so many other factors that can either make or mar us. This development leads us to a stage where we have to be concerned about our own health (both physical and mental), how we let our lives affect people around us, and the way our behavior is affecting society on a large scale.

Over 40% of U.S. adults are obese, and considering less than fifty years ago that number was one in every hundred people, the number has increased considerably in a short period of time. Apart from the U.S. being known to be one of the most vulnerable locations in the world with a substantial obesity problem compounded by culturally poor dietary habits, it is also known to have a decreasing state of happiness. In short, our state of physical health has a high impact on our state of mind, and vice versa.

As a society, we blame our health problems on a variety of institutions, such as the food industry, because they continue to manufacture products that promote obesity or are hazardous to our health. In addition, diverse cultural aspects motivate social irresponsibility and negligence. However, instead of blaming the presumed causes of this hostile situation, we should start focusing on finding a fix. Things are not getting any better in other parts of the world, which prompts the dire need for a general and natural ways of regulating and stabilizing the situation before it becomes a major health catastrophe.

As it stands, one way to correct these challenges is by establishing a strong exercise routine, taking on a proper diet, and embracing a change of approach. However, it's easier said than executed. We are no longer children; attempting to change a habit as an adult is almost the same as trying to swim against the tide. You've already been built to have certain behavioral patterns from childhood, so changing your default psychological framework can be much scarier than you thought.

Notwithstanding, if there's a will, then there is a way. Before you can change anything about your habits, you need to have a mindset that believes you have a chance at customizing your way of life. Just like Henry Ford said, "Whether you think you can or think you can't — you're right." Do you want to start making more sense of your life by living with a purpose that is different from the path you are already treading? Then start thinking you can, and you definitely will, that's the way the universe works. Although it is a very established fact that human habits from the early stages of life are imperative when it comes to development and the formation of one's life, it doesn't mean a habit is permanent and can't be modified. If you're fortunate enough to have been raised with an impressive personality and remarkable cognitive skills, then you already have a template to work with. On the contrary, if you're someone who has endured a poor childhood upbringing or experiences, then you need to focus your attention on finding a new path.

The purpose of this chapter is not to deeply explore the psychological behavior of humans, but rather to explore the relationship between your early development and your habits, physical health, and mental health as an adult, which in turn affects your relationship with the outside world. As it has been established, family, cultural background, and social norms of our environment create dietary habits that shape our foundation, and as we age, these habits become our new norms. Many times, when not properly managed, these habits can lead to poor health conditions and also have enduring negative psychological effects on our minds. When our physical body is not happy, it becomes difficult for the mind to operate in a peaceful and productive state.

Before we plunge into discussing the solution to the current problem, we need to have a clear understanding of why you've been going through your present situation. Understanding your current status will give you the chance to create a prospecting plan and build on it.

Let's divert a bit to the complications of bad early development. There are several side effects of a poor upbringing. In terms of relationships, health, and productivity, early development can have severe negative impacts on an adult. We will discuss a few of them, but you need to be aware of the following effects to compare them with your current lifestyle. This is necessary to prepare you for the new life ahead of you. Fathoming out any form of miseducation you might have had while growing up as a kid will change a lot of things, but that's the power of awareness.

Adverse Psychology Impacts of Poor Early Childhood Development

To effectively manage the future of our society, we must identify and address problems before they become uncontrollable. Biological research on stress states adverse early childhood development, such as poverty, negligence, or abuse, can weaken brain architecture development, setting the body's response system to stress on high alert permanently. Furthermore, science has also revealed that providing steady, responsive, and nurtured relationships during the earliest stages of life can avert or reverse the detrimental effects of childhood stress, which can lead to lifetime benefits such as an increase in learning and cognitive skills, a higher level of ethical behavior, and a more stabilized state of health.

The following are the impacts of early childhood experiences:

Influencing the Developing Brain

The most rapid developmental stage of the brain occurs during the first few years of life. And these early experiences will determine the fragility or sturdiness of brain architecture. During early complex stages of brain development, the circuitry of the brain is most likely to be influenced by external experiences, either good or bad. And that's just the science of it. The sensitivity of our brain during early childhood periods is very high and adaptive. Any wrong signal from external experiences can trigger a devastating, long-term effect on a child's lifestyle in the future. For instance, studies show that kids who are transferred into orphanages shortly after birth due to negligence are prone to have dramatically reduced brain activity relative to kids who have never been institutionalized.

Chronic Stress

Scientifically, our body has varieties of physiological ways of responding to threats, including an increase in blood pressure, stress hormones like cortisol, and heart rate. However, when a child has supportive relationships with adults to protect him/her from these feelings, he/she can easily learn to deal with everyday trials and challenges, leveling down the stress response system. Medical experts call this "Positive Stress." In other words, every child needs an abundance of support from adults during early childhood development.

Many adults nowadays react negatively to some situations because of one or more traumas they went through while they were younger. These traumas could be the shocking loss of someone special to them, being abused, or an unexpected natural disaster or damage. These adverse experiences have the potential of causing damaging effects on their stress hormones, causing it to rise to abnormal levels. Therapy sessions are generally recommended for adults in this kind of situation. However, there is another solution that is more therapeutic and naturally beneficial for this problem, which will be explored in another chapter.

Early Adversity Leads to Lifelong Problems

Adults who have experienced negative stress, also known as distress, during their early lives, such as destitution, physical abuse, physical neglect, emotional abuse, parental substance abuse, sexual abuse, loss of a caregiver, emotional neglect, natural disaster, mental illness, or exposure to violence, are likely to go through serious physical and psychological health problems. The more negative experiences in early life, the higher the probability of having a rough adulthood.

Various health problems can be developed from these adverse childhood experiences, including depression, anxiety disorder, disassociation, aggression or anger issues, shock, confusion, denial, muscle tension, rapid heartbeat, fatigue, lack of focus, insomnia, sudden pains and aches, addictions, and other complicated health issues.

The following behavioral disorder patterns are signs of poor childhood development:

<u>Attachment Disorders:</u> Adults who had traumatizing experiences when they were between the ages of 1 and 3 have a higher tendency to have difficulty forming and maintaining healthy attachments and relationships with the individuals they care about. This condition is often termed Reactive Attachment Disorder (RAD), which affects a person's ability to create appropriate social relationships. This disorder can impact an individual's mood and behavior. Adults with this disorder find it hard to trust other people.

Passive-Aggressive Behavior: Survivors of early childhood trauma often nurture excessive anger they can't handle. Instead of confronting and dealing with their painful emotions, they bury them deep in their conscience and allow them to keep interfering with their daily dealings. They end up developing passive-aggressive behavior that isolates them and ruins important relationships.

Inconsistent Self-Concept: This is referred to as a state whereby an individual doesn't know ways of construing personal feelings and thoughts about oneself. The inability to differentiate these perceptions and emotions causes a prejudiced and distorted view of some specific groups of individuals.

Lowered Cognitive Ability: Children who are frequently neglected or abused often develop mental snags such as memory glitches, poor communication skills, and the incapability of concentrating or focusing on tasks. This lowered cognitive ability usually continues into adulthood.

Poor Behavioral Control: Most impulsive adults are likely to have experienced some kind of childhood trauma. Most times, those who experience certain ordeals during their youth find it hard to control their behavior as they mature. So, most end up doing anything they want because they've never learned other ways to cope or they feel it's their only means of getting the attention they've been denied.

Altered States of Consciousness: Repeated childhood trauma that spreads over many years is capable of forcing children, as well as some adults, into a serious dissociative condition. It is difficult for children to identify diverse states of consciousness, so they can't prevent themselves from sliding into them. These twisted reality states cause a disconnect from their true selves and some valuable things in their lives. Even when they transition into adulthood, they tend to still rely on those delusional states for survival during stressful times.

Perpetual Victimhood: The line between good and bad is blurry to children, so it is quite impossible to comprehend the reasons bad things happen. Due to that, they often regress to illogical or absurd reasoning to justify negative occurrences in their lives, which often overflows into adulthood. Being emotionally neglected or abused forces an individual to form his or her identity in a victimhood state, and whenever that happens, it becomes quite hard to see him or herself as someone with power or control in life.

Our Current State

We can't control the occurrences of the past that led us to where we are today, which shaped our brain, programmed our cells, and switched on certain genes. Therefore, since we can't go back in time to fix our childhood, we can only plan to remedy the present to have a better future. An exciting thing about being human is you have the power to take control of your life at present. Nothing about you is fixed, not even your mindset. You have to believe you have the power to influence both your physical and psychological realities, because you do!

Viktor Frankl, the Austrian neurologist and psychiatrist, once said, "Between stimulus and response, there is a space. In that space is our power to choose our response. In our response lies our growth and our freedom." Even the perception that it is difficult to change is just a mindset. Your body and your mindset are linked. The more you improve your mental habits as you develop, the more positive feedback your body will give.

As I close this chapter, I want you to believe that you have the ability to choose how you behave and perceive things, which will modify your brain, genes, and cells.

This is a preparatory chapter to believe in yourself and make unwavering decisions from what you're going to learn in subsequent chapters. Let's move!

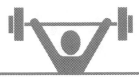

CHAPTER 2

EXERCISE AND FITNESS BENEFITS

"It is health that is real wealth and not pieces of gold or silver."

~ Mahatma Gandhi

F inally, we can start discussing the core purpose of this book. In this chapter, you will discover many things you thought you knew about exercise and fitness. Many of us believe we already know some of the benefits of exercising, even people without the education or training know these benefits.

Exercising is as old as time. In the early ages, soldiers trained their bodies every day to get more fit, physically conditioned, and skilled for combat. You can find a plethora of books that are majorly dedicated to this chapter alone.

Nevertheless, it's not the amount of knowledge that matters; it's the quality and implementation. The most efficient way to acquire new knowledge from this chapter is to put aside the old ideals and try to see beyond the norms of our understanding the topic of exercise. Let us make a breakthrough together and discover new fundamentals that can drastically enhance life in all aspects, not just physically, but psychologically and spiritually as well. Without further ado, let's dive into the business of the chapter.

The effects of exercise play a huge role in our health development and progression in life. To be explicit, let's split these benefits into two parts:

the physical benefits and the mental benefits. The fundamental idea is that the core and general benefit of exercise and fitness is the chance to improve the quality of life, and, in the long run, live a healthier life, both physically and psychologically. Now, let's start to examine some of the most important characteristics of the physical elements together.

Physical Benefits

Scientists have always tried their best to uncover all the physical benefits of exercise. Still, they always end up stating there are more physical benefits of exercising than discovered as of today. There have been several groundbreaking pieces of research that establish the positive and constructive long-term impacts of a dynamic and active lifestyle.

Medical researchers have been dazzled by the amazing things exercise does to the human body. Dr. Susan Cheng, a medical expert, once said, "I often tell my patients that if we had the ability to put what exactly exercise does for us into a pill, it would be worth a million dollars. The irony is, of course, that exercise is actually free." From facts and figures on exercise, it is safe to say that exercise is a gift from mother nature to improve our body. Below are some of the astounding ways exercise is physically beneficial to the human body.

Enhances the Body's Powerhouse

The mitochondria, the powerhouse of the cell, seems to effectively burn off more fatty fuel in active individuals. Biologically, the healthier the mitochondria, the less probable it is for an individual to develop several age-related diseases such as heart disease, diabetes, Alzheimer's, or Parkinson's. Fundamentally, one of the physical benefits of exercising is increasing the chances of an individual living healthier, specifically by enhancing the mitochondria.

Slows the Aging Process

Why do human age? Every human is programmed to go through a process of deterioration and old age. Aging occurs as a result of a variety of complex changes that transpire in our normal biological functions. These changes extend from the buildup of damage of our DNA to protein dysfunction and altered communication within cells, as well as among distant body tissues. Enough formality, this simply means we die by deteriorating.

Now, how does exercise come into play? People who exercise while younger are known to have higher life expectancies than those who do not exercise when younger. Although the reason for that is just starting to become clear to various scientists, exercise has since been linked with longer life. The biological reason for this is exercise sustains the caps (telomeres) in our chromosomes. Telomeres are known to naturally reduce as we age. However, exercising miraculously slows down the rate telomeres shorten in the body. Do you wish to have a chance at competing with Methuselah? Exercise!

Boosts Agility

This is one of the most known physical benefits of exercising. Agility simply deals with the movement of the body. Although this is mostly associated with athletes, you don't need to be an athlete to derive this benefit. Everyone wants to be able to control their bodies, make smart moves, have great reflexes, and compete with a cheetah. Some people even exercise for this alone simply because their profession depends on it, such as athletes, dancers, factory workers, soldiers, wrestlers, and the like. However, this is not only for the show; exercise ensures you have a stable core, strengthens the joints and muscles, makes you less susceptible to injuries, supports healthier bones, quickens the healing ability, reduces fatigue (energy boost), and improves coordination. Simply put, exercise gives you a higher chance of saving yourself from danger.

Supports Weight Management

For some people, there is a crucial life-threatening reason for exercising. The perseverance of obesity in different parts of the world is alarming; it's a global concern! It also has been a huge debate among healthcare professionals, as well as the government, for many years. It is fair to say the public health in the United States has a lot of room for improvement and it is in dire need for change. As good citizens, we can do a lot to help with this, for our own health, as well as our community. Whether by signing up at a gym or engaging in other frequent physical and inexpensive exercises, we can take measurable actions to improve our quality of life.

Exercise can help significantly with obesity and weight loss. When does obesity occur? Obesity takes place when a body mass index is 30 or greater, which can significantly increase the possibility of serious health problems. This is the root to many health challenges we witness.

By engaging in high intensity, or practical physical exercises, we increase our caloric expenditure and burn off excessive body fat. This formula, along with proper daily nutrition based on your body and daily activity, will help with obesity by improving the weight-loss process, reducing health risks and concerns, and improving the overall quality of life. Life is a long-term investment, so why not invest in the most precious thing—yourselves? Fortunately, obesity can be managed. It does require changes, but, believe me, it will be worth it!

Increased Energy, Brain Health, and Memory

People don't usually believe a human can have the combination of enhanced energy, ideal brain health, and sharpened memory. However, exercising shows this can be achieved in every way. With an adequate exercise routine, you can enhance your energy, brain health, and memory simultaneously! When it comes to memory and many conditions associated with it, exercise can, in fact, improve blood flow to the brain and help with memory. It also stimulates chemicals in the brain that can help boost learning, critical thinking, and overall mood.

Isn't it amazing that brains and brawn can be found in a single person? Your race and background does not matter; with a consistent exercise routine, you can be both strong and smart at the same time.

Exercise has more to offer the human body that we care to know. As it stands, it is known to balance the entire ecosystem of the body, prevent diseases, and lower cholesterol, along with many other benefits, to fight diverse common health concerns and trends in this country and other parts of the world.

Conclusively, exercise and fitness are not only known to decrease the peril of diseases, but they are likewise known for the mortality peril they confer. Plus, since many medical studies reveal that more than half of the deaths that occur globally due to cancer could be averted with frequent exercise, it is reasonable to conclude that physical exercise could significantly reduce a large number of worldwide deaths.

Mental Benefits

Although exercise plays a crucial role in the human body's system and structure, it has an even bigger role on a human's mind. There are many psychological benefits that one can gain through exercise and proper diet that can drastically improve the emotional and spiritual dimension of life. This hidden secret has not gained enough attention in the fitness world because the value of being in a good state of health, until today, has mainly been focused on physical appearance. However, most professional individuals in this field strongly support the need to sturdily focus the attention on the mental aspect of fitness and exercise.

This time around, it's not only about building muscle or an attractive physical appearance; it's more about your personal life and mental wellbeing. Biologically and psychologically, exercise enhances our brain. A healthy lifestyle improves your mood; this is generic in the sense that every benefit you get from exercising makes you feel good. You feel good when you have an attractive body, when you have great reflexes, when you have shining skin, and when you always look young and sharp, besides some other physical benefits of exercise. However, it doesn't end there; exercise, more importantly, makes you happier. When you engage in a solid exercise routine, hormones, such as endorphins, induce positive feelings, evicting negative ones. These benefits make exercising a good and genuine form of therapy, especially for individuals with mental and emotional challenges. It doesn't matter if you're a mall-walker or a marathoner, exercising helps you stay alive in more ways than you can imagine.

So, let's proceed to break down these mental benefits into fractions to be more precise. You might just be able to find the solution to what you've been struggling with for a while. Below are some of the outstanding mental benefits of exercise and fitness.

Anxiety and Depression Reduction

Anxiety is known to be one of the major causes of nervousness, fatigue, depression, or even suicide. It's a natural reaction of the body to disproportionate levels of distress, worry, and fear. Medical experts are always trying to discover the cure for anxiety, but the best way to battle it right now is with medical treatments and chemical drugs to suppress it. To be specific, there's no real cure for anxiety or depression; however, exercise does not only help reduce anxiety or relieve stress, but it also can significantly help prevent it. What's the scientific explanation? When you exercise, concentrations of your norepinephrine, a chemical in charge of moderating the brain's stress response, increases. Therefore, by exercising, you get to reduce stress, while also boosting your body's capacity to handle mental tensions.

Medical practitioners, in some recent cases, recommend patients suffering from diverse anxiety disorders join a gym center, run a few miles every morning, or just work out for an average of 30 minutes per week. This is because exercise and antidepressant pills have almost the same effect on depressed individuals.

Improves Self-Confidence

There are a lot of folks out there with low or no self-esteem. Most of them resort to disconnecting themselves from society or going to extremes to get others' attention, regardless of the means. This doesn't have to be. Basically, physical fitness and exercise can improve positive self-respect and boost confidence. Weight, gender, size, and age do not matter; you can easily elevate your perception of your self-worth by exercising. With your hard-earned sweat, you are teaching the mind the value of discipline, hard work, and dedication. Therefore, this new reality will give you a sense of pride, help you develop a stronger character, and enhance your psychological self-respect.

Do you wish to feel and look like the earth is beneath your feet? You can start by practically getting a treadmill beneath those feet to motivate yourself with daily encouraging affirmations. When you repeat saying something to yourself, and you believe in what you are saying, the mind develops a belief mechanism that can turn those declarations into actions. That's the power of affirmation!

Averts Cognitive Decline

Our brain has a way of breaking up with us as we age. I guess *"Beauty and Brain"* can't do without each other considering our beauty declines as we age, as does our brain. We can't stop the process, but exercise can significantly slow it down by propping up our brain against the mental decline that starts at about age 45. When people work out, especially those between the ages of 25 and 45, the brain chemicals that stop hippocampus degeneration become more effective. The hippocampus is a vital part of our brain that handles memory and learning. Not everyone knows this, but now that you do, at least you can start working out intentionally for a purpose.

Sharpens Memory

Does it sound weird to you that exercise could sharpen your memory? You might be asking yourself, "How does a simple 2-mile run every morning sharpen my memory? Is that not the job of a food diet, consuming stuff like eggs and milk?" Well, it's surprising, but you have to believe it because this is scientifically proven!

Regular exercise boosts an individual's memory and the ability to learn new things. Just like the previous benefit mentioned, working out increments production of hippocampus cells, which deals with memory and learning. Therefore, research has associated the brain development of children with physical fitness level. How amazing!

However, exercise-based brainpower is not just for kids alone. With a regular workout routine, an adult's memory can likewise be boosted.

Kids do a lot of running around, playing games, and getting involved in a lot of physical activities; so, no intentional physical exercise is necessarily needed for them. On the contrary, as an adult, we need to be intentional about it.

Relaxes the Body

Most people with a desperate need for relaxation look for a short-term remedy to calm them down from whatever tension or pressure they feel. They might start taking dangerous stuff like opioids, toxic prescription drugs, or other harmful substances that could endanger their health, without being cognizant of the after effects. If they only knew there was a better, long-term cure, maybe they wouldn't have unnecessarily endangered their lives.

According to scientists, exercising can also be said to be as effective as a sleeping pill. This even works on people battling insomnia. When we engage in physical exercise, our body's core temperature rises and we become hyperactive. A few hours after, when the temperature drops again back to the normal level, the body feels the need to sleep. To be able to rest, you have to work!

Controls Addiction

Dopamine, the chemical responsible for anything related to pleasure, is released by the brain anytime we do something that pleases us, such as eating food, being romantic, listening to music, meditating, and others. Sadly, some individuals get addicted to dopamine; therefore, they start depending on various substances that generate it, especially substances like drugs and alcohol. Fortunately, exercise has a lot to offer on addiction recovery.

A frequent exercise routine can effectively distract alcohol or drug addicts, defocusing them from craving the substance, at least for a short time. Simply put, when you engage in exercises, you get pumped up and occupied, de-prioritizing all forms of an alternate and depraved form of pleasure-seeking.

The list of mental benefits goes on and on, some you'll even find incorporated into subsequent chapters. By now, you should know that exercise and fitness can have amazing, positive effects that can significantly change the course of your life for good.

As we deeply discuss the benefits of exercise, start thinking of ways you can establish a solid and effective exercise routine. Look around you at what can hinder you from dedicating some time for exercise. Is it your family, your job, your friends, or your old habits? Remember, you're doing this to improve your efficiency in all these facets. Jay Cutler, a pro bodybuilder, stated, "What hurts today makes you stronger tomorrow." So, take it slow and build a better life out of it. Remember, even if you haven't found the solutions to your life challenges in all the benefits listed here, don't give up—we still have a long way to go. Brace up!

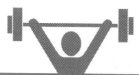

CHAPTER 3

SECRET TO THE BEST MARRIAGE WITH EXERCISE

"The difference between an ordinary marriage and an extraordinary marriage is in giving just a little 'extra' every day, as often as possible, for as long as we both shall live."

~ Fawn Weaver

You are probably questioning what exercise and marriage have in common, but hold that inquisition until the end of the chapter, then you'll have your answer. A fitness coach will tell you the physical benefits of exercising, while a medical expert will give you countless health benefits of exercising. However, a lot of what you'll read in this chapter is not information a coach or medical expert will provide; only a therapist or life coach would be willing to tell you most of what you'll find here.

Your Marriage-Exercise Future

Did you know one of the best therapeutic benefits of exercise is its effect on marriages and relationships? This has been a hidden secret, and we will investigate why together

If you're someone who is planning to create a family in the near future, and you don't want to compromise things, then carefully pay attention to every word in this chapter. If you already have a family and things seem to be falling apart, then this chapter is for you, too. Lastly, if you're someone who has a happy family but is willing to take that happiness to the next level, then this chapter is for you as well.

To begin, let's discuss a few facts about marriage status in the world. In the United States alone, there is approximately one divorce every 36 seconds, and there are about 2,400 divorces each day. Averagely, marriages that end in divorce only lasted for eight years. Lastly, the U.S. ranks 6th in the world's highest divorce rate. All these facts are enough to tag marriage failure as a national concern.

Now here's an exercise-marriage fact for you: The American Journal of Epidemiology observed the health behaviors of about 8,900 adults over many years and discovered that both men and women who married during the time of the study lost a significant amount of their cardiovascular fitness. As a couple, you don't have to carry out a study before you know that being married can derail your fitness regime. A lot of couples complain about their physical exercise life routine and being unable to balance their careers, family, marriage, and health. There's a very high chance you get disconnected from your exercise routine immediately after marriage because you have more responsibilities and duties to fulfill. However, some people don't see this as a big deal; they believe it's just part of maturing, which is wrong. Even though it may seem difficult and unreasonable to devote more time to exercise and fitness after marriage, staying fit as a married couple is a worthwhile endeavor. Research reveals that married couples who remain fit derive benefits that significantly contribute to their marriage success.

Now, exercise is not and can't be the solution to all marriage issues, but it's going to help with bonding and establishing invaluable disciplines together as a couple, like goal setting, dedicating yourself to a mutual practice, and perseverance, which all have the potential to help you battle marital fatigue. All relationships need energy and effort to be invested in them to thrive, and this is not only about struggling to make ends meet or performing duties. If strategically carried out, the impact of exercise in a relationship might just give you that happily-ever-after you've always wanted in your home. Don't forget, you have only one goal, which is twofold—to get yourself in shape, and to do it together with your partner. These two parts of your goal will ensure the effectiveness of the exercise in your marriage as well.

Without further ado, let's move on to see diverse ways exercise can mold or save a marriage.

Exercise's Magical Marriage Effect

Facilitates Teamwork

Teamwork is vital in the business world; however, it's also needed in a lot of relational platforms. It is difficult for a relationship to thrive without teamwork between partners. Teams, or couples, that carry out physical activities together build powerful bonds. If you observe well enough, you'll notice how teamwork strengthens relationships between friends, workmates, athletes, and even religious folk. Teamwork is also crucial in marriages.

How does exercise come into play here? When couples exercise together, they create a synergy that enhances their physical, mental, and emotional connection. Their bonds get stronger and infallible, making them work better together as a team. By waking up together, getting ready, and going for a run or to the gym, the sweat, pain, and soreness, the entire process, will ultimately create a very unique bond that is almost impossible to develop and duplicate through any other coupled activity. Teambuilding activities strengthen marriages by increasing trust, encouraging better communication, promoting honest engagement, solidifying a connection, and enhancing problem-solving skills, as well as many other outstanding benefits that give you the perfect home.

When interviewed, a lot of couples that exercise together speak of how working out has made them learn to better trust each other, communicate clearly, and find solutions to problems together. Isn't it exciting how much running a few miles every day can build your dream family? If you desire to run a happy home, the race literally begins now, every morning!

Builds a Powerful Household

Nothing is more powerful in creating a strong household than parents whom through their actions turn out to be role models for their children. Kids are constantly watching and observing adults, and when they see parents work hard at something with dedication and sacrifice, they begin to learn and monitor daily practices quickly, from an early age. This gives us the best opportunity to be a great role model for our kids. Once you're able to demonstrate you're a focused, empowered, and driven parent, you'll earn their respect, love, and attention much faster and more effectively.

Additionally, setting up a standard exercise routine ensures your household involves in more nutritional cooking and builds habits that are based on a healthy life routine every day. This way, you can benefit from a healthy lifestyle while also securing a healthier future for your kids. This is because they will become more familiar with eating a healthy diet with higher nutritional benefits, as well as quality organic substances rather than sugary and unhealthy substances that could negatively impact their growth process, future health, and body structure.

It doesn't stop there, though. Creating a regular exercise routine for your family ensures your kids become active at a younger age, learning from their parents, and also developing a better bond with them, just like in the example of "teamwork between couples" we discussed. Additionally, it will significantly decrease the chances of your kids developing unnatural and immoral habits such as drinking, smoking, doing drugs, or being misguided when they start maturing. Basically, a couple's workout massively contributes to building a strong, healthy, and united household.

A Couple's Happy Place

Are you familiar with the term "runner's high"? If not, it's a term that describes the euphoric feeling, reduced stress, and ability to be less sensitive to pain that an exerciser feels during a workout. All these effects are due to the massive release of endorphins during exercise. According to statistics, about 15 million adults suffer from depression, which does not bode well for relationships. Furthermore, psychologists report that depression doesn't only affect the individual suffering from it, but it also has a colossal effect on the other individual(s) in the relationship or family.

As mentioned in the previous chapter, the treatment for depression is broad since there is no permanent clinical cure. Most prescribed treatments for it are pharmacological. Therefore, many professionals in the field keep including exercising as one of the most effective means of treatment. Since it has been established that exercise treats and prevents depression, a lot of damage can be averted in relationships where emotions run high and partners react to each other because of depression. In summary, exercise facilitates a happy relationship.

Detoxifies the Body and Relationship

It's a concrete actuality that our moods are capable of affecting our relationships. Whenever our body is down, it is often reflected in our emotions. Our system needs to be cleansed to get our mind, body, and spirit in order and balance. Our body is programmed to react to almost every feeling there is in the world. There are toxins present in our bodies that make us feel wobbly; exercise offers help in clearing out of all sorts of bitterness and nightmares.

You don't have to be wholly devoted to an exercise routine; even a moderate exercise routine has constructive effects on our body. Exercise helps improve blood circulation, energizes the lymphatic system, lubricates joints, enhances digestion, strengthens our muscles, and, most importantly, removes toxins. Toxins control how we feel, which influences our relationships. With less toxins, we can feel a lot better and improve our communication aptitude.

Relieves Marital Stress

Stress and marriage are often not far from each other. As a family man or woman, you are prone to feel stressed at some points in your marriage. However, the intensity of the stress matters a lot, and this is because extreme stress can decrease marital satisfaction. We've already made a point about how exercise can help relieve stress in the preceding chapter. If you're the breadwinner of the family, stress can increase your odds of encountering unwanted, negative interactions. From job issues, family matters, heavy responsibilities, and unanticipated events, stressors can arise, and you can easily break down and start behaving unseemly towards your loved ones. For instance, studies have shown that men feel less marriage satisfaction as parental and work stress increases. This puts every couple in a position where there is a dire need for cooperation and partnership in eradicating stress instead of embracing codependency.

Energizes the Body and Relationship

The more you carry out an activity, the more comfortable and habitual it becomes. This is also the same for exercise; the more you work out, the more it becomes a norm in your daily life. As a matter of fact, adults who engage in at least twenty minutes of mild-to-moderate aerobic exercise three days per week for six consecutive weeks show increased energy levels and less fatigue. This means if an inactive person starts this type of exercise routine, their blood flow will be enhanced, allowing nutrients and oxygen to be transported effectively to muscle tissues due to the body's chemical adenosine triphosphate, which improves energy productivity.

Now, how can this save your marriage? Your energy level can determine how much you contribute to your relationship. In a marriage, there is an incessant exchange between partners. Your marriage can suffer if you refuse to invest in it. Not to mention, there is no way you can invest your heart if your body is always weak and tired. Furthermore, various medical researchers have concluded from their studies that exercise has a very high potential for enhancing sexual gratification in marriages.

This information might not be essential for unmarried couples right now. Nonetheless, you should pay attention to this if you plan on having a happily married life!

Enhances Sleep Quality

Truth be told, nobody can wake up and be in their happiest mood when they've just had a rough night. You'll understand this better if you have ever experienced prolonged nights without any sleep. When that happens, it affects your entire mood, and then your family or partner receives unpleasant treatments from you for that day.

How you start your day matters; sleep deprivation can increase emotional reactivity. Medical scientists believe individuals who struggle with sleeplessness or insomnia tend to respond negatively when they encounter a setback or disappointment. Therefore, negative reactions take an enormous toll on our relationships. One of the ways to identify a healthy marriage includes how the couple deals with challenges in proactive, positive ways.

When we react negatively to situations, it can damage our relationships. Nothing good comes from emotional edginess. Exercise assists in regulating your body, providing better rest to react in a more constructive way toward your partner.

Mutual Communication and Interaction

A relationship is about communication and interaction, not to mention that physical interaction strengthens bonds. Physical activity with a partner has a way of improving physical conditions, increasing self-esteem, increasing productivity, creating better social awareness, facilitating empathy, and, most importantly, providing a sense of belonging. Moreover, effective communication is essential in every relationship, as we all have experienced. One way to improve the techniques required and channels of communication needed is through bonding deeply and physically interacting with our partner. With a moderate physical engagement with your partner, you make ideal plans, overcome tough situations, and crack complex issues together. In summary, exercise makes you connect with your partner on a higher level

A Pleasurable Marriage

"Till death do us part" is one of the marriage vows that scares some single people to enter a relationship. If you're going to commit the rest of your life to your marriage, then you might as well want to consider having fun while at it. Exercise is fun when carried out alone, but it's even more enjoyable when you engage in it with your partner. It may not be comfortable at first, but with time and consistency, you'll include it in your list of hobbies.

Believe me when I tell you the "runner's high" feeling experienced by enthusiastic exercisers during a workout is something you want to experience with your partner. At some point, exercise becomes a habit you won't want to stop doing because the more you exercise, the more relaxed you become. The need to exercise becomes an addiction, but a good one. If you have children that you can work out with, that makes it more perfect and enjoyable. Spending family time working out together or going to the park for a family run or a bike ride can go a long way to cement your marriage and build strong family chemistry.

A lot of people think they don't need to get involved in marriage-related discussions. However, most of what we need to learn and work on in our marriages are done before the marriage. Marriage is not a testing ground; you need to prepare yourself for it while you're still single.

Exercising will give you a good head start on your marriage. Additionally, exercising can remedy a wide range of marital issues. People rarely connect the usefulness of exercise in marriage, especially its ability to create happiness and fix things.

Studies have revealed that after joint participation in a thrilling physical activity or challenge, couples feel more satisfied and relaxed with their relationships, while also falling deeper in love with their companion. Working out together can be the best form of therapy for couples. When both parties are on the same page on their diet and workouts and also living a high-quality life together, not only does it improve their overall physical health, but it also adds many more layers of profound love and trust, and a higher quality of unity and happiness as a family.

Additionally, parents become great role models for their kids, creating a better household atmosphere. In essence, the addition of one simple element to a couple's routine can be the problem solver of all obstacles in their marriage or relationship. A healthy body, a clear mind, a happy household, a great role model for the kids, a deeper state of love, and stronger communication can be achieved through exercise. Technically, exercise can be a great foundation-building mechanism for just about any relationship. You just need to look beyond the desire for it and start seeing the need for it.

Notwithstanding, the same method won't work for all marriages. There are different types of couples with different attitudes, home settings, outlooks, and cultures. There is a need for you to find out how you can introduce and incorporate exercise as a routine in your family.

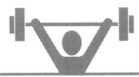

CHAPTER 4

THE IMPORTANCE OF SLEEP AND MEDITATION

"Everything you do, you'll do better with a good night's sleep."

~ Arianna Huffington

Nature requires us to sleep; that's why we have night times to ensure there are a limited number of activities we can do. Sleep is not just a period for us to visit dreamland, but it's also a phase for our body to recuperate. Meditation can also be a mechanism to bring us to this state of peace and rejuvenation. Let's discuss why we need to sleep first, and then move on to how we can get a good night's sleep, along with its importance.

Technically, you can't last for over two weeks without sleep. Some people in different parts of the world are driven by the need to achieve some spirituality goals, so they suffer their bodies by pushing it too hard. Notwithstanding, the magnitude of the aftereffects is always disastrous.

Many motivational speakers will say that great achievers don't spend all night sleeping because they are nocturnal. However, they will never tell you about the side effects of irregular sleeping. A lot of people just follow this "billionaire mentality" of making money, financial gains, and spending their nights recklessly without proper physical rest or without regard for their health. Just to ensure you know the importance of sleeping, let us discuss the constructive upsides of regular sleep and the devastating downsides of sleep deprivation.

MIND AND MUSCLE

Benefits of a Good Sleep

Catherine Darley, ND, Institute of Naturopathic Sleep Medicine in Seattle, says, "Getting enough quality sleep is critical to keeping our brains functioning well." The brain functions at its full capacity when we get a proper sleep, making a regular sleep pattern imperative.

A Healthy Heart

No doubt, this is a matter of the heart, and it shouldn't be taken lightly. The heart reacts negatively to both over-sleeping and under-sleeping. According to modern day studies, regular short sleepers have a 48% tendency to die from or develop coronary heart disease, while regular long sleepers have a 38% tendency to be exposed to this disease.

In addition, night workers and nocturnal folks who stay awake when they should be sleeping can develop heart damage. Medical scientists believe this happens as a result of a disruption in the circadian rhythms, which causes issues with biorhythms and increases stress hormone levels.

Facilitates Social Interaction and Mood

Studies have revealed that sleep deprivation can potentially reduce the ability of an individual to actively identify imperial social signals and respond to them appropriately, like recognizing and interpreting facial expressions. The body responds better when it's been given enough time to rest and recover. Just like you have to refuel or service a machine so it can give you a hundred percent functionality, your body, too, needs time to recharge itself, especially the brain.

Also, suboptimal sleep can cause mood changes, and not in a good way. Many people who sleep less experience side effects of sleep deprivation like frustration, social disconnection, irritability, and even depression symptoms. Sleep has an important part to play in the regulation of our emotions, either positive or negative, and also in the enhancement of impulsivity and productivity. Apparently, sleep deprivation lessens the ability to respond to emotional stimuli, thereby making it problematic to make exploits in our social worlds.

Lose Weight

When you maintain a healthy weight, you can avoid a lot of unnecessary health complications and be proud of your shape. But if you keep sleeping improperly, being overweight should be on your list of worries. Depriving yourself of sleep makes your body release more cortisol (stress hormone). Aside from several other adverse effects, having a high level of cortisol signals your body cells to accumulate more fat.

Furthermore, sleep deprivation triggers the release of hormones responsible for controlling appetite (Ghrelin and Leptin). This causes an individual to feel hungrier more often, making him or her feel less satisfied with every meal. And as we all know, eating a lot is a pathway that leads to obesity.

You feel tired if you don't rest, and getting tired often makes it difficult to cling to a specific diet. You just feel vindicated to "cheat" on your diet with the excuse of eating any food that improves your mood or sugary snacks that boost your energy levels. Therefore, relying on a routine sleep pattern will help regulate your body to help control your weight.

Improves Memory and Performance

For the brain to function optimally, adequate sleep is a necessity. Sleeping affects the ability to focus, solve problems, recall important information, perform outstandingly, and carry out other tasking activities.

While we sleep, our brain goes through a process called memory consolidation whereby information from the transitory short-term memory is moved to the long-term memory storage. Diverse kinds of memories consolidate at different phases of a sleep cycle; thus, too little sleep will halt this consolidation. Consequently, the lack of regular sleep patterns can alter memory storage and sorting, which can have negative effects on retention.

Lowers Inflammation

Your body does not need high levels of inflammation. When you sleep less, you increase the chances of heightening the level of inflammation within your body. Unfortunately, the more inflammation your body experiences, the higher risk of developing diabetes and heart disease. Also, inflammatory conditions like arthritis can easily penetrate.

As the popular saying goes, "Prevention is better than cure," and a good night's rest can help thwart unnecessary health complications, such as inflammation conditions.

Decreases Diabetes (Type II) Risk

One of the negative effects of irregular sleeping is the tendency to develop Type II diabetes due to how sugar is processed in your body. A study carried out on a few individuals who were allowed to only sleep for 4 hours in a night for five consecutive nights resulted in all participants experiencing a 40% decreased insulin levels; insulin is the hormone responsible for regulating the body's sugar usage. Other pieces of research reveal that under-sleeping can negatively influence glucose metabolism and lowers insulin sensitivity, raising blood sugar levels.

Enhances Physical Activeness

If you are an athlete or performer, then you should know that getting a good rest is essential before a competition or presentation. In this regard, sleeping serves the same purpose. Studies have shown that an adequate sleep routine effectively improves an individual's speed, agility, reaction time, accuracy, and productivity, especially for an athlete. That's why most athletes treasure their sleeping time, as their profession depends on it.

Moreover, sleep deprivation reduces the ability of the body to utilize glucose as a source of energy during workouts or public performances. Do you desire to be at your best state of mind and body? The resolution is to sleep to provide your body a sufficient amount of recovery time.

Boosts Immunity

Your immune system is like a soldier protecting the kingdom from being infiltrated. A weak soldier won't last long in a battle against invading enemies. You should know that many infections and diseases are always trying to penetrate your body; so, if you don't get sick often, be grateful for your strong immune system. There are many ways to build the immune system; however, one natural way to build a better immune system is to have an adequate amount of sleep. Even a little sleep deprivation can significantly decrease the rate your immune system functions, reducing its response and lowering the blood level of cells that fight off infections.

According to various studies, individuals who sleep regularly have a higher antibody count that respond to vaccinations. Therefore, if you just succumb to your body when you feel tired and sleep when you should, your body will serve you much better and you'd be less vulnerable to infections and diseases.

Cleanses the Brain

Only while we sleep can our brains flush out waste products accumulated during the day. These substances contain beta-amyloid plaques that can cause neurodegenerative disorders like Alzheimer's.

According to sleep experts, this process can only be carried out when our brains are inactive, that is, asleep. Therefore, many medical professionals believe, and it is scientifically proven, this is the prime purpose of sleep.

Increases Lifespan

Virtually every benefit previously discussed contributes to elongating our lifespans. Notwithstanding, a regular sleep routine has been independently proved to promote longevity. Studies on the effects of sleep on our lifespans have shown that individuals who sleep below 6 hours in a night are 12% more liable to die prematurely. Individuals who sleep for over 9 hours in a night are 30% more liable to die prematurely. Proper rest can contribute to the immune system, identifying harmful bacteria and viruses and thereby being able to destroy them correctly. Improper sleep patterns change the functionality of how cells work in the immune system; they can be weakened and powerless to respond and attack viruses. Consequently, you could get sick more frequently.

Considering today's world with viruses such as COVID-19, this can be a lot more impactful than just fighting the common cold. In some cases, this could be life-threatening. As we enter this day and age of unknown global developments, it would be wise to be better prepared and take preventative measures.

A balanced sleep routine is crucial; too much or too little can be hazardous to your lifespan. A good night's sleep, a healthy diet, along with proper guided meditational practices, can drastically improve the quality of our state of mind, strengthen physical state, and contribute to an overall enhanced lifecycle.

How to Sleep Effectively

Now that you know how sleep can save you from troubles such as diminished overall health, lack of energy, fatigue, difficulty concentrating, increased heart problems risk, increased anxiety and depression risk, high emotional sensitivity, less production, and so on, you might be worried about how to start sleeping effectively.

It's necessary to have the right knowledge about how to calm down and prepare to sleep, or you will just be doing what you think is right, even when it's wrong. Sleeping has different states, all which create many advantages to simply bring the mind to a peaceful state of rest, preparing it for a good, deep night's sleep. Let's look at some of the ways we can have a good night's rest.

Meditation Techniques

One of the top relaxing techniques in the world, meditation, has proved to be a very effective activity. In Eastern culture, meditation has been practiced for thousands of years with the ability to bring the body to a full state of relaxation and bliss, which is beneficial for the health of the body and mind. Meditation's importance is significant in every individual's life; by applying this ancient practice daily, you can change your life's pattern in a way that brings every other thing into balance.

Meditation produces a deep state of relaxation and effectively calms our entire biological system, which brings the mind into a state where rest and even healing can take place. Yes, you heard it right, healing! Many people with severe cases of cancer and other critical conditions have reported major improvements and, in some cases, "miracles" through the power of meditation. This shows the importance of being in a harmonious and peaceful state of mind for the two dimensions in the human anatomy—the physical state and the spiritual state.

Meditation is simple and flexible; it's a practice you can carry out anytime, anywhere. It doesn't require any tool or equipment; all you need is time. Although it might look uncoordinated at first, with time, it'll become natural and comfortable for you.

To start, before sleeping, find a quiet area (probably your bedroom), sit or lie down (whichever feels comfortable), then close your eyes. Take ten slow, deep breaths and try to clear your mind. Once you begin to feel the state of peace and calmness, simply remain in that state for a few minutes or as long as you can. Visualize being in a space with no time, no place, and no subject, just complete peace and joy. Gradually, you will feel your mind starting to clear out. You will notice a more balanced state of mindfulness. This is the state you want to sustain and remember for as long as you can. This space is the land of complete bliss and contentment.

With the help of meditation, you will experience many new changes, some will even be life-changing. In addition to all the added benefits, this new discipline will help you get to sleep faster, as well as truly get the deep sleep your body desires. For more information on the extensive benefits of meditation and how meditation can change your life, refer to my next book on meditation to be released this spring.

Regulate Light Exposure

Whatever you do, always try to limit your light exposure before bedtime. The hormone, melatonin, that is controlled by exposure to light, assists in regulating a person's sleep-wake cycle. When it's dark, your brain releases more melatonin, making you sleepy. However, when there is too much light exposure, the brain releases less melatonin.

It's safe and beneficial to be exposed to bright morning sunlight, as it helps get you active. However, you should try to avoid staring at anything too bright at night before bedtime, such as your television or phone screen. If you must use any gadget with screens before sleeping, reduce the brightness. Also, ensure your room is dark when you're about sleeping; you may keep it at the minimum brightness in case you wake up at midnight. However, you should consider that inadequate lighting can lead to frequent and prolong awakening.

Calms Your Mind

This is almost the same function of meditation. Your body doesn't respond well to sleep when it's under pressure. For instance, it's not beneficial to see a scary movie before sleeping. Getting involved in disturbing activities before bedtime can disable an individual from getting deep sleep. Maintain your stress level and get some solitude before sleeping.

To reduce stress before bed, find a soft music playlist to get you in that relaxed mood. If you've been angry with anyone during the day, try to let it go by focusing on something else. Also, don't get used to using social media or your phone when it's almost time to sleep; it keeps your brain unnecessarily active.

Maintains Your Body's Sleep-Wake Cycle

This strategy allows your body to be more energized and refreshed. Your body is like a machine; it knows when to rest and when to work. To achieve this, always try to sleep and wake up at a set time daily. Pick a bedtime and stick to it, and as time goes by you'll start waking up without an alarm. This helps optimize your sleep quality and schedule your day properly.

Also, you might want to avoid oversleeping during your leisure time, even on weekends. It can unbalance your sleep cycle, making you feel sick after. You can also recompense for late nights, but it should be done with daytime naps only, and you should be smart about how you take naps. Try as much as possible to avoid after-dinner drowsiness. When you feel sleepy before bedtime, get busy.

Eat and Drink Smartly

What you eat can determine how you sleep at night, especially an hour or two before your bedtime. Therefore, try to limit nicotine, caffeine, or other substances that can cause sleep problems. Also, ensure to avoid big meals for dinner; a heavy stomach can make it hard to sleep. This is a fact, not only for sleeping purposes, but also for your health. Medical experts suggest eating smaller meals. Avoid smoking or drinking alcohol before bedtime also; it ruins your night rest. Drink fewer liquids during the evening and reduce your sugar and refined carbs intake as well.

Engage in Daytime Exercise

As we've discussed in previous chapters, exercise can bring you to a state of relaxation and comfort. You can engage in yoga, which is great for stretching the muscles and joints. Individuals who exercise often sleep much better at night as well, and they are also very active during the day, enhancing productivity. Exercise helps insomnia symptoms, and provides a better quality of sleep.

Creates a Good Sleep Environment

Does your bedroom look like a concert stage with many lights and sounds? Then you need to make some changes. The atmosphere of your bedroom can determine your quality of sleep. Therefore, ensure to keep your bedroom cool, dark, peaceful, and quiet. Get a bed you're comfortable sleeping in. Don't bring third parties like your TV, phone, laptop, or tablet to your bedroom. Your bed is meant for good quality sleep alone.

Learn How to Go Back to Sleep

People often wake up briefly from their sleep during the night, but it's not an offense. However, if you don't find it easy to fall back to sleep after, you need to find a fix. Don't think about anything disturbing while briefly awake; just clear your thoughts and let your body naturally drift back into a state of rest. Visualize or meditate, focusing on your breathing patterns alone. This should nicely assist with a full good night's rest.

Sleeping is not rocket science; anyone can fall asleep, even in the most horrible conditions. The key to getting the proper sleep is to focus on your environment and removing the outside influences from your sleeping pattern. Create a peaceful resting place in which you concentrate on clearing your mind and allow your brain to refresh itself. As the Dalai Lama stated, "Sleep is the best meditation."

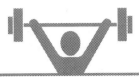

CHAPTER 5

GROUND ZERO—
WHERE TO START

"Every accomplishment starts with the decision to try."

~ John F. Kennedy

U p until this stage, we've successfully discussed so much about the usefulness and importance of a healthy lifestyle. It's high time we started discussing how you can start taking action. You already have the knowledge of how exercise and fitness can turn your life around; however, without making plans to start this life-changing routine, it'll all be pointless. Therefore, this section will give all the ideas and knowledge you need to start the journey.

Remember, exercise is a lifetime journey, so how you start matters a great deal. If you've been asking yourself how to kickstart this exercise lifestyle without complicating things in your environment, then you need to pay close attention to the instructions in this section.

The first thing you need to know is you will have to make sacrifices along the way. As previously discussed, it's not easy to change a habit due to our early development factor; therefore, expect many obstacles and resistance from your body, mind, and even your family or loved ones during the process.

As the famous quote by Lao Tso goes, "A journey of a thousand miles begins with a single step." Don't expect to build a new healthy lifestyle in just a few weeks; it's almost impractical. Instead, trust the process and ease into it; after all, Rome wasn't built in a day either. You'll be frustrated a lot of time along the way, wishing you had never started, but that's quite normal. Consistency is the key. Many people have trodden this path and gave up halfway through. The most important thing to remember is not to give up, and that's why you need a very strong determination that will sustain you through this journey. You have to prepare your mind before you proceed with this chapter. This is because whatever you read from here on won't sound achievable if your mind is still unprepared to commit to new changes.

Before we start talking about various routine options you have for building a healthy lifestyle, we need to strategize a starting place based on the kind of life you are living right now and the one you want to adopt, and the possible sacrifices you might have to make. You have to consider several factors attached to your life. No one has the same life routine because we all have different jobs, diverse work hours, distinct family types and household settings, as well as personal life choices and many other factors that determine how our lives are structured. This confirms there is a need for a stage of diagnosis of your personal life and a plan to abide by.

Adopting a New Healthy Lifestyle

Now, you may actually already have a very decent lifestyle and a standard home setting. However, since you are incorporating something new into your lifestyle, you still need to be flexible to follow certain rules that come with the new routine. The following are some of the prerequisites of this new lifestyle.

Define Your New Lifestyle

Exercising might be uncharted territory for you before now; thus, you might want to fully define and comprehend what you're getting yourself into. It is imperative to know the sole purpose of starting a healthy routine and the reasons and goals before you commit to it. I have many friends who started out well on an exercise routine, but as time went on, they began slowing down and retreating. When I asked them their reasons for retracting, they told me they couldn't keep up with other priorities that kept popping in. I knew the reason was they just didn't commit to the routine; it was just a side activity to them. You don't get what you wish for by just sitting around—you have to work for it. Great achievers have purposes, the rest have wishes. Like Bryant H. McGill said, "Having a sense of purpose is having a sense of self. A course to plot is a destination to hope for." You have to define your purpose for exercising, dieting, and living differently. Starting a new healthy lifestyle requires you to accept becoming a different person, perhaps becoming a better version of yourself.

Eradicate Redundant Activities and Schedules

We have daily tasks and goals, and some people even have a prioritized to-do list for each day. However, to start a new healthy routine, you might need to review that list. We won't know some activities are unnecessary until we find other important activities to replace them. You have to sever all attachments with events, habits, and even thoughts that have not contributed to your ideal lifestyle. If you always wake up very early in the morning to watch TV or go through random social media updates, then it's time to postpone or completely let go of them.

Set Practicable Goals

People who set up goals to exercise and see obvious physical changes in a very short time always end up injuring themselves; excessive exercise can do more harm than good. Set feasible and achievable goals and keep track of them. Don't be too hasty to start seeing results; focus on being consistent with the routine and the goals will be achieved before you know it. Nobody can be conscious of their physical growth. They just realize one day they're big and old enough to do some things. The same goes for exercise; the expected results slip in without announcement.

Involve Your Loved Ones

When you're in a relationship, a sudden change in schedule might not go well with your partner or family. You need to consider them when making your lifestyle changes. Although the new exercise routine might require you to sacrifice some of the time you spend with them, ensure you balance it one way or another. You may choose to include them in this new healthy lifestyle you're aiming for since they might be interested in changing their lifestyles, too.

Expect Disappointments

Keep your success expectations moderate. You may encounter a few challenges, failures, and letdowns along the way. However, when you're already prepared for it, these disappointments will make you stronger and more committed instead of slowing you down. Your ability to recover quickly after a flop will go a long way to ensure you reach your ultimate goals, so endorse and welcome the pain and challenge.

The New Lifestyle

We are here! This chapter is dedicated to starting to live a healthy lifestyle. Since your mind and environment are now ready to adopt new things, it's time to initiate a new healthy exercise routine.

Create a Daily Exercise Time

Early morning exercise is the most effective exercise routine, and it works for almost everyone, working-class or not. It is recommended to wake up early so other daily schedules are not affected. This also requires that you go to sleep early. For instance, if you leave home for work by 7:30 am every morning, it's best you wake up about an hour and 30 minutes earlier, work out for about 30 to 45 minutes (it could be a few miles run or home exercises), and prepare for the day with the remaining time. This exercise routine will make you feel fresher, more energetic, and less likely to encounter stress at work throughout the day. Furthermore, according to medical facts, the body's hormones are in their best state in the early morning. This also allows you to burn more fat since you are most likely on an empty stomach or semi-empty stomach in the morning. However, I believe a light and nutritious breakfast is best practice, especially for high intensity exercise or weight training programs. Considering morning exercise is one of the most effective routines, if you are not able to exercise in the morning due to schedule difficulties, then set a time in the evening that you can commit to and make sure you fully dedicate to that time every day.

Setup a Healthy Diet

Good nutrition also plays a vital role in living a healthy lifestyle, and the only effective way to ensure a good eating routine is to be on a diet. Dieting requires adhering to a food category for a very long time. There are over a hundred different kinds of diets. Choose a diet that will serve you a lot of benefits regarding the new lifestyle you're creating. You'll still learn how to choose a diet that best works for us in subsequent chapters.

Additionally, choosing a diet might require some sacrifices, especially if you have a family. Also, you might have to stop eating your favorite food or be less specific about the type of food you cook. You have to handle this part smartly, depending on your home situation.

Manage Your Stress Levels

Stress can take you to dark corners you don't intend to go. Stressed people tend to have trouble focusing and thinking straight. Therefore, try as much as possible to manage your stress levels. You can develop a routine that ensures you minimize all stressors around you, making you feel more relaxed and pressure-free. This will give you a clear mind and enhance your ability to make ideal decisions. Whenever you are in a situation that can potentially raise your stress level, take deep breaths, and calmly think about ways to control the situation and stay focused on your goal.

Stress can come in two forms: psychological or physical. When you worry or think too hard, your mind becomes stressed and clouded; this could be from your family or social connections. When you work too hard, your body becomes weakened and stressed; this could be from your job. You have to develop the aptitude to control both situations; it's the only way to ensure a healthier lifestyle.

Create an Ideal Sleep Routine

A poor sleeping routine can ruin your entire day, and that's not a good example of a healthy lifestyle. Therefore, create a fixed sleep-wake cycle that will ensure your body gets all the rest it wants. This will constantly enhance productivity, giving you the chance to be at your best anywhere, anytime. If the new sleep routine requires you to let go of some things you love doing, such as seeing your favorite nighttime tv episodes, chatting with friends who stay up late, or playing your favorite online game, then either adjust the timing for these things or let them go. You can't just create a new, better lifestyle out of the blue without paying a little price.

Make Friends with Mutual Health Goals

This is not only about peer-pressure; the kind of friends you keep can determine how you live. If your friends tat share the same goals as you, you have a better chance of achieving them faster. Friends can be a good source of motivation when we feel like quitting. Therefore, ensure you keep friends who are on the same mission as you. It won't be easy for you to stop sleeping late, smoking, doing drugs, drinking, or eating uncontrollably if you have friends that do all these. Notwithstanding, if you have friends you can influence to join you on your quest, then don't let them go. This will be extensively discussed in the next chapter.

Join a Health-Focused Community

This goes a long way to help you develop a healthy lifestyle faster. Just like support groups, a health-focused community will get you motivated and encourage you to see the positive side of the new lifestyle and pursue it.

It doesn't have to be a physical community; there are many online communities or groups you can join that have the same goals you're chasing. There are even several phone apps built for this purpose, such as body-building apps, meditating apps, dieting apps, and weight management apps. These apps help you to keep track of different routines.

Moreover, these communities share ideas, demonstrations, testimonies, and other inspiring aspects, making it interactive and engaging.

Regular Medical Checkups

You can't possibly know your full health status by simply observing physical changes. You need to have medical checkups often to assess your body's strengths and weaknesses. Without regular medical checkups, you risk jeopardizing and complicating your body's functions. Without knowing the activities that are harmful to your body and those that are beneficial, you just keep doing them ignorantly.

You should also note that you don't necessarily have to go for checkups only when you feel sick. You can feel healthy and still have internal failing body organs. Preventative measures can go a long way. Simply put, regular medical checkups save your body from impending dangers.

Self-Control and Perseverance

Discipline is key when it comes to making noticeable changes to a way of living. Virtually every task involved in the new lifestyle you're pursuing requires a commitment. You'll be tempted to go back to your old habits several times along the way. However, consistency, persistence, and discipline will get you to your destination.

If the road to attaining a life goal was smooth, then discipline might not be needed; however, no one can promise an easy journey. Many times, you might want to slack on your diet, sleep a little later than usual, watch a few more episodes, or wake up too lazy to exercise, and that is normal to feel all those things; you can expect them once in a while. However, the primary goal is not to yield to any of them.

Take Timeouts

"All work and no play makes Jack a dull boy." Though this proverb might sound like a cliché, it isn't, as you'll only be promoting stress if you keep working your body to attain your goals without a break. Taking timeouts allows us to take a step back and refresh our body and mind. There are no shortcuts to success; the lifestyle you're trying to build takes a lifetime to complete, which is why it's called a "lifestyle" and not just a "style." Hence, take it slow and steady, build your life around it, and celebrate every victory.

Embrace All Changes

Even though the process may look inconvenient and problematic, the earlier you start accepting the changes, the faster you get used to them. Every change you make may have a certain impact on your life, either positive or negative; however, it's your job to try to balance it all out. Most importantly, you should never allow your new, healthier lifestyle to hinder important things in your life. You shouldn't damage your relationship or hurt your loved ones in the name of building a new lifestyle; it's not worth it! Instead, look for ways to personally make all the sacrifices alone; always remember that you're doing this to be a better person.

There's an inspiring quote by David Goggins that says, "Don't stop when you're tired; stop when you're done." At the end of it all, the success will be worth the pain. Never be discouraged or give up on your goals; give it all you've got. No one gets anywhere in life without being able to set their mind on a desired path and sacrifice for a higher purpose. A healthy lifestyle and the decision to "live it, breathe it" really makes a huge impact on one's life in many areas; it's a life-changing decision. So, go out there and be an inspiration to all individuals who want to make something better out of their lives.

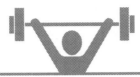

CHAPTER 6

ATTAINING GOALS
WITHOUT OBSTACLES

*"The first step towards getting somewhere is to decide
that you are not going to stay where you are."*

~ J. P. Morgan

R ead the chapter title again; it's impossible to achieve a goal without an obstacle since every goal comes with a fair share of obstacles. Some are just bigger than the others. However, your ability to manage these obstacles will determine how significant their impact will be on your goals. In this chapter, we're going to discuss how to deal with major obstacles that can affect your goals. It will be divided into two sections: how you can deal with your old habits, and how to deal with negative people and distractions.

Most times, negative people and our habits are the major interrupters of our life goals. Nonetheless, these two factors can be dealt with if you have the proper mindset and focus. You shouldn't fight a battle on two fronts, as the odds may not be in your favor. Fighting your old habits is a battle that transpires within you, while negative people and distractions stand as the battle outside your walls. It's best you choose your battlegrounds wisely.

Dealing with Old Habits

Your habits can either help you achieve your goals or ruin them. If your habits don't support your goals, you'll greatly struggle to attain them. Great achievers are known for their distinct habits. The reason many of us struggle so much to pursue a goal is our foundational habits keep getting in the way. Creating a new lifestyle of fitness and exercise demands your habits agree with your routines. Let's look at some habits that can hinder you from getting to where you want to be.

Poor Dieting

If you grew up eating anything you like at any time, it could be quite hard to change that behavior. Plus, even if you tried, there is a higher probability that the routine won't last long. You need enough determination to change this.

In the fitness world, you can't keep exercising and still eat any way you want. You need a sustainable diet that will complement your exercise results. Rich and cultured people, as well as athletes, always take their meal and mealtime seriously. You won't see them opting for fast food or junk food. They don't only eat to satiate their hunger, but rather to keep their bodies in good health and shape and to perform at a higher level.

Poor Hygiene

Poor hygiene is one of the habits of individuals who live carelessly. Educated and guided people understand that poor hygiene only paves the way for infections and diseases, thereby jeopardizing their health status. The new lifestyle you want to build is a neat one. If you're someone who doesn't care to take a shower or clean up immediately after exercising, then that healthy lifestyle you are dreaming of and working towards might remain a dream for a long time. You need to live clean to live healthy. Apart from the medical complications involved, poor hygiene can really reduce your self-esteem, affect your attitude, and give off negative vibes to people around you.

Poor Commitment Aptitude

If you are used to running away from responsibilities that require devotion and commitment, it's time to change that attitude. Exercising every morning, dieting, good hygiene, and other life-changing activities require a high level of commitment to maintain. Your level of commitment may not be 100% perfect at first, but with time and consistency, you'll build your commitment skills. Moreover, these skills will help you in so many other areas of your life.

Low Mentality

Poor perception of things can really stand as an obstacle to achieving your goals. This issue might be due to poor early childhood development, but you can reverse that ideal. You should start thinking about expanding your horizons, and even making room for more educational opportunities. Be open-minded and learn new things every day. Read books that will contribute to your level of sophistication. Move with people who are very urbane, well-versed, and polished. This will help open your mind and improve your mentality about important things like fitness and exercise, thereby speeding up your progress.

Poor Control Skills

If you are not in control of a situation, you'll barely be able to make steady and lasting decisions. For example, if you decide to start exercising every morning and you still want to text your friend or keep chatting with your partner at the same time, then you're a long way from achieving the task at hand. Put your goals first and let people know you for who you are and the decisions you make. You can't please everyone at the same time. Start being decisive, purposeful, and strong-willed. With that, you can start having things your way and work with your plans.

Low Endurance

Your endurance level has an impact on your level of consistency. If you're someone who easily gives up on things that look too tiring and challenging, you might not go far to accomplish anything tangible. Building your endurance and fortitude levels is paramount when it comes to making life changes. For example, waking up early every day to exercise, dealing with negative people, and eating foods you don't like require endurance to cope with these situations. Endurance is not easy to build, especially if you have been living your life before without having to endure much. However, if you are determined enough, your endurance level will skyrocket as time goes on.

Emotional Instability

Breaking down easily when failure strikes is a habit you need to purge. You could have developed this due to a traumatic childhood experience, but you have to find a way to overcome it. This is something that can cripple your progress. If you are emotionally unstable, you'll barely be able to think straight when an emotional situation arises. You'll be disposed to make wrong decisions and act unreasonably. Although this is one of the problems that can be solved by exercising, you still need to be emotionally stable to some extent.

Obstinacy

This is different from being decisive or purposeful; it's a state of being wrongheaded and careless. If you are close-minded and adamant to useful instructions and directives, it may be hard to secure a better future. People will be unwilling to offer their help or work with you, and your productivity level will be low. You need to have a good, attractive personality to achieve much. You have to start expanding your circle, which requires you to meet people and socialize. Obstinacy won't get you anywhere.

There are so many other habits that can hinder your progress in building a healthy lifestyle. You need to figure out the ones you are exhibiting.

Negative People and Distractions

Negative people are always known to be pessimistic and exhausting. If you are not watchful enough, they might drag you down into their mess, sidelining your goals and disrupting your focus. Let's look at a few ways to handle negativity from people.

Know Your Worth

People will weigh you according to your standard. Once they perceive you have a lesser or same standard with them, they start putting themselves in a position to control and criticize you. However, if you always look confident and poised, it'll make them feel unworthy to even give you advice. That doesn't mean you shouldn't seek advice from people; you just have to know who to approach. Ensure that person has high standards in line with your plans and can influence you positively. Don't allow negative people who haven't achieved the kind of goal you are chasing to poison your ambitions.

Stand by Your Decisions

If you don't look poised about your goals, other people will gladly recommend their own objectives to you, whether they are productive or not. You can't feed on every piece of advice and opinion people give you; instead, start learning how to remain committed to your decisions. When people impart their own beliefs, weigh it according to your goal standards, not theirs. For instance, if you have someone who always tells you to quit working out in the morning and exercise in the evening instead, look at the person and deduce if that idea has really worked for him/her. If it hasn't been working and you find your plan more effective for you, then stick to your decision and work out in the morning. Negative people often find it hard to influence people who stand by their own decisions.

Set Boundaries

Always ignore the pressure to give attention to negative people. If you keep feeding on their idea contributions, their negative energy is going to contaminate your life, affecting your attitude and goals. Therefore, set limits on how much people can influence and access you generally. If you observe that someone is presenting a negative vibe, keep your distance from him or her.

Whenever you find yourself conversing with a negative individual, ensure you shorten that interaction and excuse yourself. The human mind is flexible; the right amount of persuasion can easily influence it. You might not be able to control or avoid negative people, but you can choose whether or not to listen to them.

Disregard Complainers

Individuals who complain a lot about everything have lesser chances of succeeding in life. They have nothing to offer you to improve your life. These types of people do not offer solutions to problems, but are good at pointing them out. Listening to them will only get you invited to their pity party. You should stop socializing with friends, colleagues, or simply people who display typical grumbler symptoms. Limit interaction to a need-be basis. Build your circle around positive people with problem-solving skills.

Focus on the Important Things

Do you have friends who always try to get you involved in things they want to do? You need to reduce your interaction with them. If you don't, your goals will fade out soon enough, and you'll end up fulfilling their goals instead. You have to condense all the hangouts, partying, and other activities that don't bring you any closer to achieving your goals. Also, if you engage in pleasurable, materialistic things that consume your time, money, and energy, it's high time you started refocusing all these resources to achieve your goals.

Be Discreet About Your Plans

According to research scientist Dipanjan Das, "Don't tell your plans to anyone; just make it happen." People respect and admire results, not plans. Therefore, only tell your plans to those you must. You can carry your partner or loved ones along with your plans mainly if you know it can affect them in any way. However, aside from your close inner circle, keep third parties out of it; they often find faults with your plan and try to discourage you from executing it. Don't think you always need people to assess your plans; it's your life plan, not a business plan. Nonetheless, if you feel you can't do it alone, you can show your plans to people of value who can contribute significantly to your goals. If possible, carefully choose a mentor and carry only him or her along.

Track Your Goals

Tracking your goals gives you a sense of accomplishment, thereby encouraging you to progress with them. You can create a goal list and cross each of them off as you complete them. This way, any intruders looking to distort your goal plans will be a rare occurrence due to your mission and vision.

In order to achieve this, have a timeline of expected progress and what needs to be done. Then once the goal is reached, you can set another goal for yourself. If you are finding it hard to achieve a certain goal, don't cancel or skip it, but, instead, find another means of achieving it, either by lowering the expected result or exploring other reasonable techniques. This keeps negative setbacks off your list of concerns, giving you a clear mind to only focus on progress and completing your targeted goals.

Dominate (Be in Control)

Nothing feels better than having a sense of control, especially to prevent giving attention to deleterious vibes or irritators. You won't have to argue points with anyone if you are in control because your opinion of everything will be regarded as the best.

In the journey of building a healthier lifestyle, you'll be required to make a lot of decisions that can't be made by anyone else other then you. Some of these decisions might be complex and problematic. For instance, when you have to decide whether or not to join your friends at a late-night party when you have a gym session the next morning.

Another example would be someone who is in a rehabilitation program for alcoholism and he walks by a bar one day. What would happen if he, even for a split second, contemplates or is gravitated to the bar to get a drink? Yes, you guess it right, as soon as he accepts that first drink, the whole process of rehabilitation and recuperating is ruined. This is where the principle of being "laser-focused" plays a major role. It is very important to stay committed to your game plan. Even the slightest distraction or wrong turn can impact your end results.

The benefits of fitness are unlimited. There are always higher physical and mental levels you can push yourself to reach. Even if one reaches the stage in which they do not want to improve anymore, the goal then becomes to simply sustain the improvements. Therefore, changing old, bad habits and getting rid of activities and patterns that can mentally and physically affect one's health are critical and necessary.

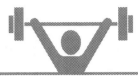

CHAPTER 7

DIETING

*"Start where you are. Use what you have.
Do what you can."*

~ Arthur Ashe

Dieting is an excellent indicator of a healthy lifestyle. However, it's not good enough to just diet; getting on the right diet is essential. Many people often wonder what kind of nutritional program will perfectly suit their body system. Some seek the advice of medical experts or nutritionists for the best diet for their body and condition, and others carry out their research and select one with noticeable benefits. There are different goals for every kind of diet. Being on the wrong diet affects your body as well as your life goals, so let's discuss how dieting can secure a better future for you as well as the right kind of diet for you.

There is a vital need to have a balanced diet plan in order to succeed with your final health goal. Diet and a balanced diet are not the same. A balanced diet must agree with your physical and mental states. What you eat is how you feel, how you feel is what you think, and what you think determines who you become. The value of good food can't be underrated when it comes to a healthy lifestyle, fitness, and exercise.

What Is a Balanced Diet?

People embark on a balanced diet for different reasons, as diets serve many purposes. You need to define your purpose for a balanced diet because without knowing why might not be effective or productive. Notwithstanding, if you still can't find any general reason to go on a balanced diet, the following are some of its prime benefits.

Promotes a Harmonious and Healthy Lifestyle

Generally speaking, a balanced, varied, and adequate diet plays an important role in instigating a healthy lifestyle. When you are hale and hearty, you have more reasons to be happy. This is one of the major reasons people diet. You can achieve happiness by simply eating in a premeditated manner. Depending on the diet you opt for, it may not contain your favorite or tasty foods, but you'll feel better and also have a very agile and strong body to flaunt. Moreover, this works well with your exercise routine since the benefits you get from your diet allows your exercise to be easier and more effective.

Boosts Immunity

Most diets involve the intake of minerals and vitamins, which help to boost your immune system. The more you adhere your diet, the less vulnerable you will be to infectious diseases. Furthermore, a healthy diet protects the body against various types of noncommunicable diseases like diabetes, skeletal conditions, some kinds of cancer, and cardiovascular diseases. A balanced diet is recommended to people who are looking to cure a disease or any medical condition; however, a balanced diet doesn't only treat these medical conditions, it also prevents them. This will be very helpful in securing a new, healthier lifestyle by ruling out health issues on your list of worries.

Manages Body Weight

Obesity is generally known to be a national problem. However, being overweight is not the only health threat, as being underweight has been proving to be a significant medical concern as well. People with underweight problems are always strongly recommended to take on a certain type of diet; the same goes for individuals with overweight issues. In short, there are a variety of diets designed by medical experts for different purposes. You need to find one that works for your health goals. The perfect diet that aligns with our goals in this book will be explained in the next section.

Calories are a great determinant of body weight. A report from the National Heart, Lung, and Blood Institute states, "A diet containing 1,200 to 1,500 daily calories is suitable for most women who are trying to lose weight safely. A diet with 1,500 to 1,800 daily calories is appropriate for most men who are trying to shed excess pounds."

Widens Your Food Experience

Committing to a diet means you are highly likely to encounter foods you've never heard of or ate before. You might need to start cooking new delicacies with different techniques. Therefore, dieting expands your knowledge about foods, giving you the opportunity to experiment with various foods from diverse cultures and origins. You can make it fun! Moreover, dieting gets you emotionally involved with foods in a good way, since as you eat different foods you are exposed to different ingredients, colors, and tastes.

There are several other benefits of a balanced diet. Every standard diet is expected to deliver the purpose it was fashioned to deliver. Athletes, singers, dancers, businesspersons, royals, and many other individuals in various fields have their balanced diets to keep them operational and productive. Let's move on to discover the kind of diet you need for your aspiring lifestyle.

The Right Diet

The meal plan about to be discussed is purposefully recommended for this book's focus only. It's a major decisive part of living a healthy lifestyle. The quantity of food required depends on your age, gender, weight, and level of activity. Calories are burned based on the kind of workout you do and its intensity. Enhancing your exercise performance through a proper, balanced diet is not only about choosing one food over another, but also about consuming the right food at the right time.

Breakfast is a very important meal you shouldn't miss, especially when you have exercise on your to-do list for the day. Regular breakfast can help reduce several medical risks like heart disease, ulcers, diabetes, and obesity. It can also help in replenishing your body's blood sugar, which is needed to power the brain and muscles. Exercising on an empty stomach when you wake up can exhaust all your stored-up energy. Even if you don't have a cooked meal ready for you before your exercise period, you can try eating some fruits to raise your energy level.

However, apart from the need to eat breakfast regularly, the content of the meal also matters. It's essential to divide your calories between three main classes of nutrients: carbohydrates, proteins, and fats.

Carbohydrates: The body breaks down carbohydrates (composing of sugars and starches) into glucose, and then later uses it as energy by the muscles. The tissues and liver store excess carbs as glycogen, and they release it as needed by the body. Glycogen is responsible for providing the energy needed for high-intensity workouts and lengthened endurance. You can get quality carbohydrates from whole-grain cereals and bread, rice, vegetables, fruit, and pasta. Nancy Cohen, a professor specializing in nutrition, reported, "By eating carbohydrate-rich foods that are low in fat and low or moderate in protein, you can make sure you have enough muscle glycogen as fuel for your physical activity. This might include low-fat granola bars, fig bars, a peanut butter and jelly sandwich, banana, yogurt, pasta, or other high-carbohydrate foods."

Protein: Protein plays a significant role in balancing your diet because it helps slow down the intake of carbohydrates, especially if you're an athlete or attempting to build your muscles. Our muscles need to be fully operational when we exercise since they become stretched through muscle hypertrophy. Timely protein intake, especially after working out, helps repair the muscles that were stressed during exercise and also build those muscles further. Examples of good sources of protein are fish, chicken, beans, eggs, tofu, and meat. For example, three ounces of chicken per meal (which equates to about twenty-four grams of lean protein) should be sufficient for the average person. Generally, anywhere between twenty to forty grams of protein is ideal, depending on your body type and fitness goals.

I always find it best practice to write down your plan with measured daily calories intake. This food journal will save you a lot of time and turn all your hard work into measurable results. It might take a little time to put together a sufficient meal plan the very first time, but your one-time investment will go a long way!

Fats: Some fat intake is also needed in your diet. Fats offers your body adequate fuel necessary to last longer during low-to-moderate exercise. Fats also support cell growth, as well as helping the body absorb nutrients to produce important hormones. Choosing healthy fats, such as avocados, nuts, and olive oil, is the important factor! When you exercise with high-intensity, where carbohydrate (glycogen) serves as the primary fuel source, your body still needs fat in order to access the stored-up carbohydrate. Therefore, having a satisfactory fat intake diet is key. For instance, if your diet is based on 2,000-calories-a-day, your objective range of total fat should be between 40 to 80 grams a day. Within that total number of fats, your saturated fat should not be any more than 20 to 25 grams. Paying attention to proper fat intake is actually a very important part of a diet, yet is most often ignored.

Water: The mother of it all! Water is essential to factor in fluids when you're drawing up a diet routine for a healthy lifestyle. Drinking enough fluids throughout the day before, during, and after exercising is very important, especially if you are someone who engages in strenuous exercise. Drink water every time you're about to put your muscles into use, even when you're at the office in front of your computer or you're not feeling thirsty. Drink water because it has so many magical benefits.

A sufficient amount of water is essential for digestion and helps avoid constipation. When you stay hydrated, you help reduce substantial toxins from the body. Another important role of drinking water, especially for obesity, is that extra water can also aid with weight loss, boost your metabolism, and cleanse body waste.

There is also a lot of research that shows the benefits of consuming hot water as well. Drinking a cup of hot water may help to increase blood circulation through the arteries and veins. Blood circulation in the body is one of the most important topics from a medical perspective. When there is effective blood flow, we can see health benefits such as improved blood pressure and a decreased risk of heart disease.

Overall, whether it's for daily purposes, sports, or the medicinal, drinking water is a topic that needs more spotlight, especially considering the fact that recent research states close to 75% of Americans do not drink enough water. Thus, the best strategy is to develop a ritual of carrying a bottle of water with you at all times. This is something I have personally found to be very useful, effective, and a wonderful habit.

Water is an essential choice for several activities. Though there are other choices, not every drink is for every lifestyle. There are sports drinks you can have before exercising, especially those that contain carbohydrates and electrolytes. However, you should know that sports drinks aren't designed for everyone; essentially, they are only for those involved in activities that require prolonged endurance. There are also drinks that cause dehydrating to the body like coffee, soda, alcohol, and tea. It is reasonable to drink the same or more amount of water as the dehydrating beverage you take.

Greens: Fruits and Vegetables

Last but not least, greens! Greens are the body's magical beneficiary! Greens are high in vitamins, minerals, fiber, and antioxidants, as well as provide folate, which is a B vitamin that provides heart health. The more research the scientific world discovers, the more we learn the importance of an herbal regime rich in natural greens, such as vegetables. Some of the best sources of green vegetables are kale, broccoli, spinach, spirulina, chlorella, asparagus, avocado, and beetroots. Recently, I have personally been consuming a lot of celery, which I enjoy very much. Celery is considered a superfood, and is a known anti-oxidant and also removes toxins, wastes, as well as contaminants from the body. Another notable benefit includes protecting the kidneys and preventing kidney diseases—and that is just one green! Imagine what benefits you would receive with a diet rich in greens.

Since it's often difficult to intake all the greens we are supposed to consume on a daily basis, I have found green fruit and vegetable powders to be very effective. They are low in calories, yet high in minerals and vitamins like vitamin K, iodine, selenium, vitamins A and C, magnesium, iron, and, most importantly, it's rich antioxidants defend our cells against free radicals.

In summary, a proper intake of greens and other unique superfoods is one of the most important elements to a strong and effective long-term foundation for one's health. It's best practice to make superfoods a priority in your daily diet.

Nutrition

Nutrition can determine the quality of your new healthy lifestyle. If you plan on creating a hyperactive exercise routine, or you simply want to improve your overall diet, you should consider eating a meal that is rich in carbohydrates, protein, good fats, and most importantly lots of greens.

For a decent and healthy breakfast, you can have a cereal rich in fiber (like oatmeal or another whole-grain cereal) combined with a low-fat dairy product and fruit or juice, or you can keep it more simplified with egg whites. You can also make a delicious protein shake with all your green and vegetable powders previously discussed, or preferably fresh fruit smoothies. This way you instantly start your day on a good note.

For lunch, you can opt for a sandwich with lean meat like fish or poultry on a loaf of whole-grain bread, combined with fruit and raw veggies. Another meal idea is veggies, like broccoli and asparagus, with a lean source of protein like tuna or tofu.

Notwithstanding, you shouldn't use protein and other energy bars as a form of meal replacement, even though they can be useful. Be specific with your bars though; only eat bars when you cannot have real food. I have seen a lot of diets that are centered around protein bars without an adequate source of real foods like greens, and vegetables. Remember, the goal is long-term health, it is not a sprint, it's a marathon.

Keto or Vegan?

At this point, you may still be wondering what works best—keto or vegan? Both are important, but the key is a precise balance. Fruits, greens, meat, vegetables, grains, super foods, and other commonly purchased organic foods are necessary for a sound exercise routine. Everybody needs to find the routine that best works for their body, as there is no "one size fits all" in this regard.

You do not need to go to extremes and completely give up on meat and your favorite foods; there are ways to get the best of both worlds. I personally find a diet that consists of 70-80% vegan and 20-30% meat (keto) sufficient to keep you healthy and well-balanced, which I call the 70/30 rule. It is centered around a balanced "happy mind, happy body" approach, as we desire a total equilibrium in our different lifestyles. As someone who has been active all his life, I have observed and discovered that a good balance of the 70/30 rule is overall the most suitable and sustainable in the long run. This way, you do not get burned out and you still enjoy life as well.

Even though you know what to eat and when to eat it, you still need to ensure you are able to make it a routine. Eating unsteadily won't give you the ideal result you expect. Most people ditch a healthy diet plan just because they do not see early results. However, it's not only about eating and seeing results, but it's more about doing it right with long-term consistency. If you observe that it won't be easy for you to take on a healthy diet all alone, then you can persuade other people in your circle to join you, or simply surround yourself with individuals or communities that are supportive.

Remember, you have control over what you put in your body, and since your diet is the most important component of a healthy lifestyle, take it seriously and believe in your long-term goal of a healthy body and healthy mind.

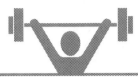

CHAPTER 8

BODY AND MIND

"When mind, body, and spirit are in harmony,
happiness is a natural result."

~ Deepak Chopra

One of the remarkable accomplishments a human can ever achieve in a lifetime is to be able to connect the body and mind into one dimension. A lot of principles are applied to this concept. From the beginning of time, humans have always tried to bring the mind and body to a state of balance. Many religions and spiritual practices have a platform for this. Monks, for instance, believe they can achieve a spiritual balance by spending days and months meditating and remaining in a state of tranquility. However, our focus is not the spiritual aspect (although that will be the focal point of my upcoming book focusing on the principles of meditation), but on learning how to integrate our body and mind to enhance our physical and mental health altogether. The body works best when in alliance with the mind. You can see the body as a ship being controlled by a small rudder, which is the mind. The physical size and shape of our body is irrelevant; it is the capacity and efficiency of our minds that are very imperial to our growth.

Eva Selhub, an internationally known medical expert, carried out a study on this subject, and stated, "In mind-body medicine, the mind and body are not seen as separately functioning entities, but as one functioning unit. The mind and emotions are viewed as influencing the body, as the body, in turn, influences the mind and emotions." Psychologists have always argued the reason the body-mind conception is vital to psychology. Notwithstanding, nature and science have always established that the body has a strong, unfathomed connection with the mind. The theory was birthed through the notion that our physical conditions effect our mental health, and vice versa. Relatively speaking, only a few individuals have been able to explore this sphere. Unlike dreams or desires, our emotions and thoughts don't exist only in our minds. Feelings are believed to be actual and physical. For example, you might have heard a lot of people say they have butterflies in their stomach when they are experiencing an emotional sensation like love or affection. Also, people who get angry easily are basically characterized as "hot-headed." Feelings of depression can also be tagged as a physical pain manifesting on a basic neurochemical level.

Your ability to function as well as your physical health is controlled by your body. For instance, simple actions such as walking and movements of body parts all hinge on the well-being of your body. On the other hand, your mind serves as a house to your spirit and drives you to function effectively.

There are a variety of studies confirming the association between physical and mental health, as well as their ultimate association with our inner energies. This integration permits our emotions, both positive and negative, to physically impact our body.

Emotions have different representations in our bodies. Let's analyze the major emotions and the body's response to them.

Happiness: This emotion fills the entire body with activity; it focuses all attention to a physical sense of readiness and heightens the communication between our body and mind. There's always a sense of security when we are in a happy state.

Love: This emotion stands out as one of the top emotions that fully activates the whole body. Love and physical desire are often intertwined; therefore, it is known to activate sensations all through our reproductive organs more than happiness.

Pride: This emotion fills the head as well as the chest with a highly intense sensation. It makes us focus on ourselves and nothing else. Pride acts similarly to surprise, as it prepares our body to confront danger.

Fear: This has an understated body activation pattern relative to rest. The body prepares to either engage in a fight or escape. However, it doesn't necessarily seek outright conflict. Fear requires the body to be alert and also prompts the brain to engage in spontaneous thinking, allowing quick decisions to be made.

Anxiety: This activates long-term, substandard stress. The chest is intensely stimulated, leading to a possible feeling of dread or doom. It has almost an equivalent experience with panic attacks, as the chest is always involved in both cases.

Apart from these five emotions, there are other feelings that alleviate the activity level of the body, such as depression, shame, contempt, and disgust. The human body is continually subjected to constant internal and external stressors that can be interpreted as the body sending messages to the brain.

Now, how do fitness and exercise help integrate our mind and body? Let's find out. There are different techniques used to achieve the body-mind integration. These approaches are meant to regulate the body's stress response systems so that equilibrium can be sustained and maintained. Scientifically, it's explained as the restoration of our prefrontal cortex activity, which reduces amygdala activity and reinstates the regular activity of our nervous system. In the medical field, there are diverse alternative methods that aim at increasing awareness and strengthening the body-mind link. These modalities include exercise, meditation, relaxation, mindfulness, yoga, and biofeedback. Let's take a more in depth look at these.

Exercise

The neurons or nerve cells in the brain make use of chemicals called neurotransmitters as a means of communication. The exciting part is that strenuous exercise increases the levels of two vital chemicals, the glutamate and the gamma-aminobutyric acid (GABA), which several pieces of research have been carried out to prove this fact. This indicates that exercise can improve communication between nerve cells and can also be a good form of therapy for depression treatment. Moreover, it has been established that exercise can improve memory and brain health as we age.

Meditation

Conventionally, the major pivotal point of meditation is the attention on breathing patterns; the focus is to breathe in and out through our noses. Various studies on meditation have revealed that being attuned to your breathing and paying attention to it can naturally slow your breathing pace. This assists the body in relaxing, lowering the chances of depression, anxiety disorder, and anger. It is confirmed that meditating for three minutes can calm a stressed brain, but on average, 5 minutes meditation is recommended per day.

Relaxation

There are different times in our lives when we are stressed by being in a state of alertness. In this state, it's necessary for us to find a means of relaxing our body so as to prevent significant damages. This is different from meditation.

Most people always have their ways of relaxing when they are too stressed. Some have favorite cool spots to visit, others hang out with their friends, and some play games or watch movies; however, if you want to really help your body relax in the most effective way, you should try a relaxation therapy called Progressive Muscle Relaxation (PMR).

PMR is a technique known to improve body intelligence. It involves the systematic pulling and releasing of muscles, dealing with a group of muscles at a time. In practice, you tense a group of muscles as you breath in, hold the tension briefly and then release the muscles back to neutral. This process helps reduce physical tension and stress by increasing the body's focus. It is recommended to practice Progressive Muscle Relaxation exercise 10-20 minutes a day. There are also other relaxation procedures you can adopt, such as Body Scan, which is often performed in the begging of mindful mediation. It helps with tuning the body and connecting the physical state to the inner dimension. Scanning helps to bring awareness to the entire body.

Mindfulness

Practicing mindfulness is a very effective tool in treating psychological health disorders, cancer, cardiovascular conditions, and stress-related conditions. Individuals who are disposed to anxiety, depression, and other stress-related conditions habitually overthink and ruminate unnecessarily. They find it hard to detach from their worries and thoughts, which is capable of driving an individual to exhaustion. Mindfulness is a good way to direct your attention to the moment's experience.

Self-regulation can be achieved through this means, and once the body feels the mind is aware of its status, it calms down. Mindfulness is all about redirecting your attention to your environment so as to escape pain, discomfort, and negative thoughts. When you disrupt your past thought patterns, your heart rate decreases and your breathing regulates, essentially relaxing the body and causing a rush of pleasant neurotransmitters throughout the body. In short, mindfulness establishes a positive feedback loop, evading the negative thoughts.

Yoga

Yoga focuses on making use of body movements to draw an individual's attention to the present. Technically speaking, the slow and steady movements are responsible for relaxing and decreasing physical stress. Negative emotions are also eliminated when in this focused and relaxed state of mind.

Biofeedback

One of the major techniques used for enhancing body intelligence is biofeedback. It involves using electrodes to measure the physiological and scientific monitoring of the body to augment the body's consciousness.

Medical experts strongly support biofeedback as a potential solution to many physical conditions. It is known to reduce some particular disorders like migraines and high blood pressure. One of its most recognized benefits is providing an individual a sense of self-direction. Biofeedback can also help with chronic ailments such as headaches, pelvic pain, asthma, sleep disorders, and recurring abdominal pain.

Most of these techniques can be achieved by creating a daily practice routine. You can make use of visualization techniques, giving clear instructions to your brain on what next to do. Also, you could start making positive associations to help visualize the positive side of things, helping to adjust your attitude in an ideal way. Lastly, you should always try to stay in the moment. The mind is prone to often drift away from the moment, being entangled in all sorts of random and unreasonable thoughts. This can be detrimental to your exercise routine. Be actively present at all moments by paying close attention to your body's feelings and activities.

The body and the mind are the most effective tools we own to attain a positive well-being. Therefore, it is important to know about body intelligence and utilize it as a side treatment and circumvention of mental and physical illnesses. You should know that activating the natural hardwiring existing in your body and mind is a perfect way to shoot your exercise up to a higher level; just keep thinking positively. Jim Rohn couldn't have expressed it better when he said, "Take care of your body. It's the only place you have to live."

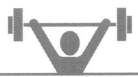

CHAPTER 9

BEST WORKOUT PLAN

"Today I will do what others won't, so tomorrow
I can accomplish what others can't."

~ Jerry Rice

I t's time to start learning workout procedures. Whether you are doing it for bodybuilding or body transformation, physically and mentally you need a perfect workout routine that fits into your dream lifestyle. You should note not all routines are for everyone; what works for your friend might not work for you, and vice versa. If you want to ensure you won't hurt your body during the exercise process, you need to find an exercise routine that agrees with your body's needs and limitations.

No one can ever give you a workout routine that is going to magically transform you into an ideal physique competitor instantaneously. It requires years of exertions and hard work; you'll experience a lot of trials and errors before you can achieve your physique prospect. The recommendations in this book about ideal exercise routines, effective sets-and-reps schemes, as well as training techniques will all work based on your mindset.

When setting up your workout routine, consider the following: workout experience, personal goals, availability, rest and recovery plan, and weaknesses. Let's explore these concepts.

Workout Experience

Beginners don't need a high-intensity workout routine, but rather a high-frequency workout routine. If you have not exercised before, you should stick to the beginner stage, and if you're acquainted with casual exercises, you may move on to the intermediate level. However, you should not skip to the advanced level until you build your way there.

Personal Goals

By now, your desired goals should be well planned out. The general purpose is to build a healthy lifestyle through fitness and exercise. However, you can have side goals, like shape management or larger-scale physique changes, that are additional to your overall exercise goals. Whatever your goals, prioritize them and make them count.

Availability

Every exercise routine requires commitment; you should ask yourself if you can consistently exercise five days a week or if your schedule is too tight to afford making time for working out for a few days a week, especially if you're a businessperson with so many random and unplanned appointments. Whatever your schedule, you should know that each workout builds upon your previous one. Therefore, you have to be ready to make use of your exercise program no less than three days a week.

Rest and Recovery Plan

Your current lifestyle, job, and recovery abilities are factors to be considered while setting up your routine. Your rest routine shouldn't be taken for granted because of your fitness aspirations. You should learn how to pay attention to the messages your body is passing across. Incorporate your rest hours or days into your new lifestyle plans.

Weaknesses

Lastly, you should know your elastic limit (also known as the yield point), the greatest limit your muscles can stretch before straining them. You should only exercise when you're in your best form. You shouldn't workout when you're supposed to be at the hospital for a checkup. You can always create another training session to make up for skipped sessions.

The main concepts to consider before starting your exercise program are essential. Now let's discuss the workout plan.

Split Body Parts Workout

To start, I'm going to list some core workouts and a split body part routine. Most professional bodybuilders utilize a split body parts program in which they focus on one part of the body at a time. This allows you to get more out of each muscle, conserve energy for your next exercise, and not lose muscle fibers due to overtraining. A lot of HIIT (high-intensity interval training) workouts these days tend to drain-out individuals, which can lead to major injuries. It is a good exercise, occasionally, or at least for someone who is already in an extremely competitive athletic shape, but for most people that is not the case. Therefore, implementing a split body part workout routine is an ideal strategy. Four to five days a week of workout is enough with the remaining days to rest.

I'll go ahead to introduce a four-day exercise routine that I personally enjoy and recommend. You can utilize this plan or incorporate it into your current workout routine. You can change the order every couple of months to shock the body, but these classic exercises have been utilized by some of the greatest athletes and are considered classic routines. Adopting these exercises will make positive and significant changes in your physical and mental health, if performed properly. In order to get the best result and avoid injuries, always warm up properly and focus on form and muscle contraction versus the amount of weight. Keep in mind, the focus is muscle and mind connection

Note: All exercises listed below should be done with three sets and ten to fifteen reps per each exercise, except otherwise noted. These exercises are some of the most important fundamental workouts for most body types. It is recommended you select the ones that are the best fit for your current condition.

Day One: Chest and Back

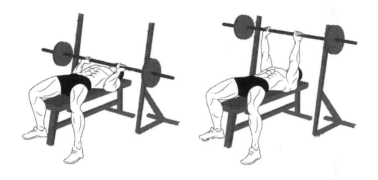

Barbell Bench Press: This drill involves the pressing of the upper body. It is commonly used for building body strength, body size, and muscle size. This movement targets muscles in the upper body, including the chest and triceps. To perform this exercise, you'll need a straight and smooth bench to lie flat on, which enables you to improve your muscle stability as well as your ability to lift heavy objects. Remember, don't focus on the amount of weight, focus on proper form and maintaining full control instead.

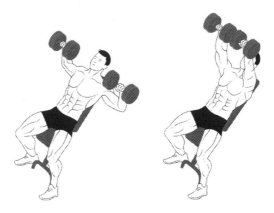

Incline Dumbbell Press: This drill also targets your chest and triceps, and it helps build a well-balanced chest musculature. It is beneficial for boosting circulation and blood flow towards the chest that can stimulate the well-being condition of the heart. To perform this exercise, get an adjustable or incline bench and a pair of dumbbells (preferable lighter than the ones you would use when you perform a leveled or flat dumbbell press). You may adjust the bench to incline about 30 degrees or a little more as long as it is a perfect angle for you. Don't use too much weight or twist your wrists; lift the dumbbells at equal intervals (don't bounce them off your chest to gain momentum).

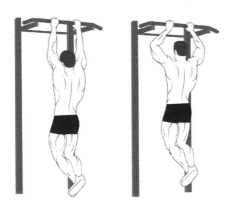

Pull-up: You can perform this exercise in a free form using your own body weight, smith machine, or using an assisted pull-up machine, which can help carry some of your weight. You can choose the type of pull-up and the level of difficulty depending on your current fitness state. This majorly focuses on your upper body to build your strength. It involves a closed-chain movement. It is a position whereby your body gets suspended and pulled up at intervals by your hands. Ensure your legs are always in a bent position when doing this so as to reduce the body drag.

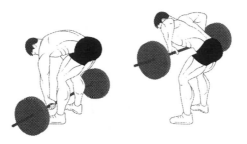

Pendlay Row: This is a form of barbell row. Make sure you keep your core tight by inhaling/exhaling with full control a few times to get oxygen levels in the core ready for the exercise. Basically, keep your abs as tight as you can. Performing this exercise will effectively build your back muscles and body mass. This can drastically help with your back posture, especially lower back pain due to poor posture at the office for hours. You can start by placing the bar on the floor and then bending forward with hinged hips and a paralleled back to lift it to the chest and back; this process counts for a rep.

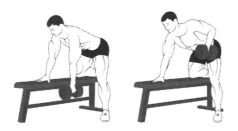

One-arm Dumbbell Row: This is a form of the dumbbell row that helps you build your back muscles. You perform this by standing with one dumbbell held neutrally in one hand, hinging forward with your torso parallel with the floor, then pulling the dumbbell close to your upper body.

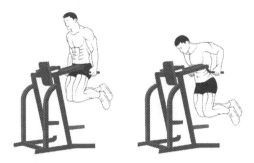

Chest Dips: This focuses on building your upper-body strength, chest muscles, and triceps. To perform this, find a parallel bar or furniture that fits, and use your hands to suspend your body. Hold your body above the bars at the length of your arms, lower your body down slowly, and lift it back up to the starting position. Breathe in when you lower your body and breath out when you're pulling back up. You can find training equipment that is designed for this at the gym.

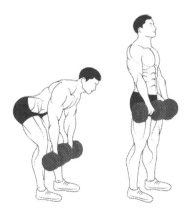

Deadlifts: This is regarded as a powerlifting exercise that can increase core strength and stability. Deadlifts stimulate both lower and upper body, with the concentration on the legs, lower back, and core. One of the reasons we have bad postures is due to a weak back and core muscles. A consistent routine of deadlift exercise will, in fact, improve posture and help with alignment and configuration of the spine, as well as other important zones. When you can sit or stand straight, you naturally breath better, and when you breath better you have more oxygen flowing to the brain, heart, and the entire body. As you can see, they are all interconnected.

Day Two: Shoulders and Arms (Biceps)

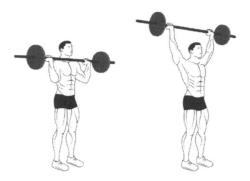

Barbell Military Press: The shoulder muscle has three groups of fibers, starting with the anterior, lateral, and posterior. Barbell military press is foundational when it comes to shoulders. This is the same process as the barbell press except it requires you to bring your feet close together, like a soldier at attention. This helps build your shoulders and core muscles.

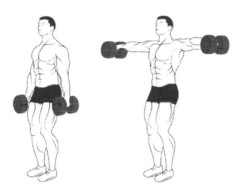

Dumbbell Side Laterals: This involves the lateral raising of your dumbbells to build developed shoulders and deltoids. It's not as simple as it seems, but you'll find it very effective in strengthening the muscles in your upper arms, neck, and back. Personal recommendation: use light weight and increase repetition for this exercise.

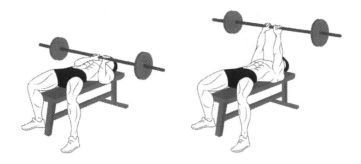

Close Grip Bench Press: This is a compound exercise of the upper body focusing on the triceps muscles; it also involves the secondary muscles, which are your shoulders and your chest. It enables you to lift heavier loads and gain maximum strength. This is one of my personal favorite movements.

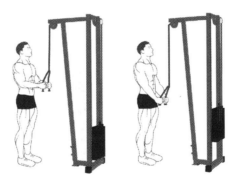

Rope Pushdown: This is a very common exercise that targets the triceps muscles; it also regarded to be very easy to perform, making it a lot of people's favorite. Try to keep your elbows close to your body, while bending your knees marginally and keeping your back as straight as possible the entire time. Three sets and ten reps per routine is recommended for this exercise.

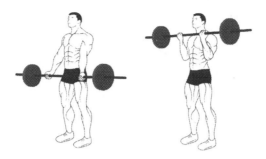

Barbell Biceps Curl: This exercise involves standing and holding the bar at the thigh level, squeeze, and with full focus on the biceps, lift the bar to the chest and back down. Three sets and six to eight reps per routine is recommended for this exercise. Level of difficulty and the "how much weight" factor should always be: first set is the lightest at 20-40% of your power; second set lift about 60-70% of your total power; and your third set can be your heaviest set, of course while being able to keep the proper form as discussed earlier. This methodology can be applied to most exercises.

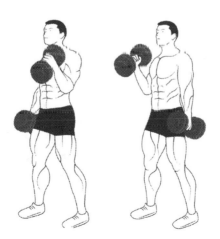

Dumbbell Hammer Curl: This helps build your bicep muscles. To perform this, stand with your feet shoulder-wide apart (not too wide), slightly bend your knees while your elbows are kept close to the body, and curl your dumbbell to your shoulders, squeezing your biceps for a second, then slowly lower the weights. You need two dumbbells to perform this exercise. Three sets and six reps per routine is recommended.

Day Three: Legs and Abs

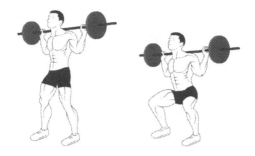

Barbell Squats: This focuses on weight training for building the strength of your legs and abs, and it also has long-term health benefits. To perform this, start by setting up the bar and the rack properly, and then bend your hips and knees together to lower your body while keeping your heels even with the floor. Push your body back up and repeat from the start position. Four sets and eight to ten reps per routine is recommended. For men, this helps to release free testosterone and growth hormones with anti-aging effects in the body. For women, besides working on better posture, it helps muscle definition, toning the glutes, and prevents cellulite formation. This exercise in a way is the mother of all exercises.

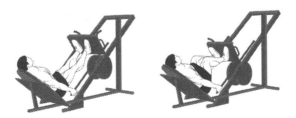

Leg Press: This is quite a popular exercise. There is a machine available for this at almost every gym. It helps build the quadriceps and gluteus, as well as the hamstrings. It is important not to lift too much weight. Start by raising the head and hold your breaths, shorten the motion range by placing the hands on the knees and sit properly when performing this exercise. Three sets and ten reps per routine is recommended.

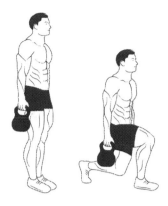

Walking Lunges: This is just the opposite of the static lunge. The difference is you won't have to stand back upright immediately after you perform a lunge with one leg; instead, you take a short forward movement with another leg by lunging it out. This exercise strengthens your leg and core muscles, glutes, and hips. Three sets and six reps per routine is recommended.

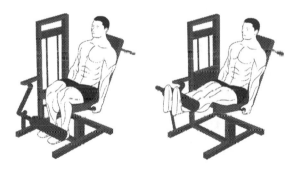

Leg Extensions: This is a weight training exercise that involves resistance. It focuses on building the quadriceps muscles. There are various types of leg extension machines designed for this purpose. Three sets and twelve reps per routine is recommended.

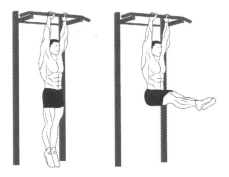

Hanging Leg Raises: This exercise is quite advanced and only recommended for major exercisers. This helps flex the hip and abdominal muscles. It involves hanging by your arms on a bar and raising your legs above the ground in a parallel form. Four sets and ten reps per routine is recommended.

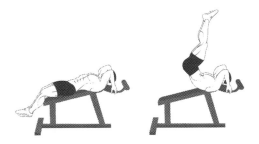

Dragon Flags: This exercise is also advanced and not recommended for casual exercisers. It helps build legs, abs, and core strengths. Start with your hands in a fixed overhead position by gripping the sides of the bench. Tighten your torso and lift your legs up into a reverse crunch. With your body rigid from your shoulders to toes, slowly lower your legs in a controlled motion without letting any part of your body touch the bench other than the upper back and shoulder. Then lower your body until it hovers over the bench. Four sets and five reps per routine is recommended.

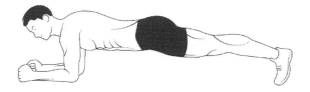

Planks: This is an exercise for building overall core strength. It involves remaining in a body position similar to a push-up stance for a period of time. Four sets with one minute each is recommended.

Day Four: HIIT and Cardio

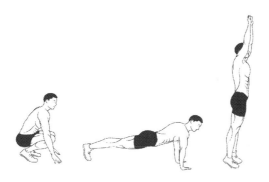

Burpees: This is known as a full exercise that puts the entire body in an active state; it is also known to be an aerobic workout and used for building strength while burning lots of fat and calories. It's an up-and-down movement like a push-up and then a jump that involves stretching the arms and legs and bending the hips.

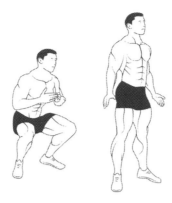

Squat Jumps: This is considered a power move. Your thigh and butt muscles are needed to propel your body up and support your landing. The quads, calves, hamstrings, glutes, and other lower-body muscles are tested in this exercise.

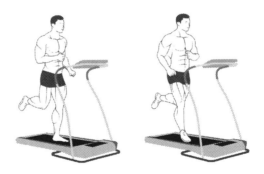

Running/Sprinting on a Treadmill: Using the treadmill or running a few miles does a lot more than pumping your heart; it puts your entire body in an active state, helps you lose weight faster, improves heart health, improves muscle tone, and improves sensitivity. Twenty minutes of running is recommended per routine. You can add couple of more exercises such as elliptical or cycling bike to your cardio day if you desire. The main idea on your cardio day is to not go over an hour of high intensity training in order to sustain maximum muscle energy for your next workout.

Weight Training

What is more important, weight training or cardio? Both are necessary. Your primary focus is to attain a good balance of both.

Weight training is one of the most important elements of your success. Weights will help you develop more muscle mass, burn more calories (if done correctly), and also give you a sense of developing "strength." The sense of having this power and energy is due to the repetition of lifting weights consistently, so you naturally become stronger as you progress. The progress of mentally knowing that you can pick up a 25 or 85 pound dumbbell, for example, gives you a good feeling of strength, power, and concentration. The journey of weight training gives an individual a sense of pride, joy, and boldness, resulting in an improved overall state of health that leads to a great psychological effect as well.

On the other hand, cardio has its own way of increasing your heart rate, strengthening your heart muscles, boosting your mood by generating endorphins (a good-feeling chemical that is released by the brain), reducing arthritis pain and stiffness because of joint movement, and helping to sleep better. So, a good combination of both weights and cardio in moderation is the key.

There are several other forms of effective exercise that can give you the desired results. Some of these exercises might even be your favorite sport or hobby. You can engage in aerobic exercises such as jogging, playing tennis, climbing stairs, dancing, swimming, biking/cycling, and multiple others to build your endurance. Most of the exercises previously discussed are for strength building, which is also very effective for building a healthy lifestyle.

If you want to engage in flexibility exercises that will enhance your reflexes and give you full control of your body, you should start considering incorporating yoga, Pilates, and other exercises that involve stretching several parts of your body. Likewise, if you want to obtain body balance, try exercises like standing on a foot, heel-to-toe walking, and practicing tai-chi stances.

However, you should be careful about the kind of training you adopt and how frequently you do them. As a beginner, you should stick to the basics for now; your body will signal you when it's time to advance to the next level. People who prematurely take on exercise routines done by high-intensity exercisers, runners, swimmers, boxers, wrestlers, competitive builders, and many other professional athletes always end up injuring themselves. Also, people who are hasty to have a perfect body structure usually push too hard, which leads to negative results and even injury. Ensure to balance your workout routine, and your workout will definitely work out.

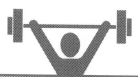

CHAPTER 10

PSYCHOLOGY AND FITNESS

*"The muscle and the mind must become one.
One without the other is zero."*

~ Lee Henry

In this chapter, the imperceptible relationship between the mind and muscles will be considered. It's going to enlighten you on some powerful relationships between psychology and fitness, both scientifically and conventionally. Understanding the connection between them can go a long way to expand your horizons and exploits in the fitness world.

As you age, your body and mind transform and are often expected to get weaker; however, they can also grow stronger in some ways. For example, constantly putting your mind to work by learning new things and engaging in mind-challenging activities like solving puzzles and mysteries keeps your synapsis in tune. The same goes for your muscles; constantly tuning and challenging them as you grow can help you enhance your strength and fitness, which, in turn, helps you avert possible future defects, such as being easily susceptible to injuries. It's simple logic.

Notwithstanding, there's a big connection that exists between the body and the mind. The more attention you give to building your physical strength, the more your mind is going to be tuned to everything going on with each part of your body. This way, you'll develop the ability to continuously challenge both your body and mind. For example, when you visualize and direct all of your focus to each muscle you're training during a workout, your mind can better communicate with your body to perform that exercise effectively.

We can simply refer to the muscle-mind connection as a deliberate and conscious muscle contraction; it creates a clear difference between actively and passively performing an exercise. Whenever you concentrate on making use of a specific muscle to create contraction, your brain employs a higher percentage of muscle fibers in that region to finish the task. Your brain's ability to focus on a particular action for a specified amount of time is called "Focused Attention." In this regard, there are two types of focused attentions needed during a workout: internal focus and external focus. Let's look at the differences between these.

Internal Focus: This is when someone focuses on the details of what goes on *in the body*. For instance, when performing a crunch, the mind concentrates on contracting all the muscles in your anterior abdominal while also flexing your spine.

External Focus: This is how sensitive someone is to his/her *environment* during a workout. For instance, when you're on a leg-press machine, your external focus should be on pushing the platform with your feet, away from the torso.

Even though both focuses help improve performance, studies have revealed that internal focus contributes more to muscle development and growth. Therefore, if you wish to enhance your muscle-mind connection, concentrate on all the muscles that are needed to lift the weight.

To consolidate your body and mind during exercise, ensure to do the following:

Select Cues

You shouldn't work on more than a single cue at the same time. Fitness trainers and coaches make use of cueing as a tool to help improve their clients' activeness and performance. As an exerciser, you can also personally make use of cueing to develop the way your brain links with the correct muscle fibers. Concentrate on your form and breathing to ensure you note precisely what you desire to achieve.

After producing some cues, try them one by one. The first and most important cue is to have a proper setup. If you completely focus on your setup pattern, your brain will register it as your default setup. You solidify your muscle-mind connection faster when you concentrate on movements individually instead of trying to learn everything at once.

Tension Building

According to fitness experts, the time spent under tension when going through resistance training serves as a vital component for building muscles. Your muscles increase in size and strength when you spend more time lifting weights under tension. You can increase your time under tension in several ways. One of these ways is to take a short pause during maximum contraction. For instance, when performing a glute squeeze, you may hold it when you get to the highest part of the bridge, pause at a flexed position when performing a biceps curl, or maintain your position at the lowest level of a hand push-up.

Slowing down the eccentric or elongated part of a workout is another way to build tension. Adding about three seconds of eccentric movement enhances your muscle-mind connection. The reason is your mind reflexively concentrates on being in control of the slowed-down movement. Isometric contractions are also an effective way to increment your time under tension; this is because it promotes your brain-muscle relationship. Examples of exercises that work for this are planks, iso-hold squats, and isometric chin-ups.

Eliminate Distractions

The belief that humans have the ability to multitask is a misconception, and this is not about rubbing your belly while patting your head. Your workout gets easier when you focus your attention on the gains instead of the pain. Additionally, turning off distractions, such as your television and phone, enables the brain to concentrate on the current task. Music is known to be an effective way of energizing your body when working out, but it might be best to leave podcasts and audiobooks for the treadmill session. Your presence at the gym should only be focused on you, the weight, your movement, and your muscles, with no other outside distraction.

In summary, the mind has numerous ways of connecting with the muscles when working out. Select something to concentrate on for a particular period, and you'll become more attuned to your body's frequency. If you are not used to exercise, it might be best to begin by removing all unnecessary distractions around you. Moreover, the best method you can use to build muscles faster is by incorporating eccentric contractions in your exercise. If you're already a gym expert, concentrate on isometric and concentric contractions and build some cues into your exercise drills to activate your concealed muscle-building potential.

Life is a gift, so is our body. After all, we are just the tenant of this house for a countable number of years, so why not construct it and make it beautiful?

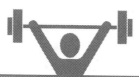

CHAPTER 11

REACHING OUR GOAL

"Discipline is the bridge between goals and accomplishment."

~ Jim Rohn

Yay! We're finally here. Even if the journey wasn't as smooth as you expected, you made it! Now that you've been reborn, you have almost everything you need to make a difference in your life. It's time to start a new day, a new chapter, and a new lifestyle. However, since you've successfully set up a good routine and understood all the values of a healthy lifestyle, how do you stay consistent and focused? Don't expect things to flow smoothly or you'll be disappointed.

Setting up a lifestyle is not the real achievement, but the key is to maintain it. You need to have a certain level of mental preparation to sustain the set routines. In this chapter, we're going to look at how we can make sure we keep doing what we started without getting tired or giving up.

You have enough motivation needed to be interested in this new lifestyle. We've spent several chapters discussing the benefits of a healthy lifestyle. What you need now is discipline, and a lot of it. Everyone can set goals, form a plan, and even get started; however, it takes discipline and dedication to sustain all that feeling of excitement about the potential outcomes of the lifestyle.

You may feel you don't really need much discipline because you think you're strong-willed enough, but, trust me, everyone feels that rush of excitement and determination at first. But once you start facing different obstacles and hits from every angle, it will be as though you made a mistake embarking on that journey. Ever wonder why a lot of people are so passionate and motivated to attain this kind of lifestyle, and yet they don't make it beyond two weeks of consistent workouts and healthy meals? Do you regard it as laziness or incapability to live a fit life? No, it's not laziness or incapability; it's all contingent on the level of discipline. Notwithstanding, you don't naturally become disciplined; it takes a lot of time and practice to develop a moderate discipline level.

In this regard, you need self-discipline to achieve your goals; you need to have the ability to make decisions independently and control yourself. It's a self-commitment that requires you to always follow through with your plans. There are over a thousand things we would rather do with our morning than rise early at 5am to exercise, even if it's just to go right back to sleep. Nevertheless, there are those who take bold steps of setting their alarm, getting up, and completing the workout. Simply put, discipline is when you commit to something and follow through. Motivation only involves feelings and reasons, but discipline involves action and devotion.

Here are some of the ways you can stay on the new path you've chosen.

Stop Making Excuses

Excuses and discipline are enemies. Even though many excuses are often valid, they still hinder us from reaching our full potential. If you want to stick to your goals, you have to avoid making excuses as much as possible.

You can begin by ensuring you start your day early. This way, even if you have an infinite to-do list, you can, at least, maximize those extra hours to make a difference.

Furthermore, you need to learn to make both long-term and short-term plans. As Benjamin Franklin said, "If you fail to plan, you are planning to fail." Not knowing what you want to do, as well as the right time to do it, will only keep generating excuses. If possible, assemble your plan into phases, from phase 1 through phase 11 with different categories of objectives; this way, they become more attainable. This will also help keep things on track more effectively.

Additionally, you should always treat your workout session like an important daily appointment; let it always be part of your schedule. If you must, even send yourself a calendar invite. Know the type of exercise you're performing each day and the time allotted for it.

Know Your Purpose

Even though awareness of purpose only serves as a means of motivation, it also has an essential role to play in building discipline. Motivation may not last, but recall it's an aspect of discipline. Being confident about your purpose of exercising will help you during times when you feel low. All you have to do is look back and remember why you started to help drive you when things are not looking promising.

Be Realistic

Everyone already has so much happening in their lives; we are almost always busy. We sometimes find it hard to create time for ourselves. Therefore, this calls for you to always be genuine and realistic about your journey. Know what's attainable and what's not in order to ensure you don't end up ruining or unbalancing other important activities in your life. If you're always busy with work or other necessary duties, look for adjustments you can make or activities with lesser priorities that you can eliminate. For instance, if you're a night-shift worker and you always spend your morning sleeping because of a sleepless night, schedule your training session around the afternoon or evening time.

It takes time to build self-discipline. You're not expected to be perfect from the onset. However, you need to have a mindset that allows growth and improvement in aptitudes. Learn from every mistake, and don't stay down when you fall, and always work towards perfection. If you get tired at some point in your journey, seek support from professional trainers or get a workout partner.

Expect to be opposed by some individuals who aren't interested in your goals. There'll always be obstacles and barriers on your way, and the more intense they become, the closer you are to accomplishing your goals. If you've learned one thing from this chapter, it's that your future lies in your hands. The level of effort you put into this new responsibility will determine whether or not you'll go far. Fix your eyes on your goals, regardless of the storm you'll face on the way. It'll definitely be worth it in the end.

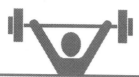

CHAPTER 12

MISSION ACCOMPLISHED

"Be the hero of your own story.
Show the world the quality of your character, the strength of
your resolve and the size of your heart by finishing strong."

~ Gary Ryan Blair

At this junction, it's safe to say the purpose of this book has been fulfilled; our mission is accomplished. Together, we've successfully transversed through many life-changing processes that can, hopefully, contribute to a more balanced and healthier lifestyle for you, both physically as well as spiritually. If you're reading this chapter right now, you have probably started the process of planning. Hopefully, a new you has been born, and you are not the person you were when you started reading this book. With any luck, this book has helped you increase your levels of frequency, and, without a doubt, believing in the power of yourself. Most importantly, you've taken some bold decisions with measured preparation that will change your life. Even though this chapter draws the curtain on the book, it's the beginning of the road for you.

So far, so good. In this book, we've been able to cover all aspects of a healthy lifestyle. We now know how much fitness and exercise can positively change physical and mental health, prevent diseases, improve the quality of relationships, strengthen family bonds, improve married life, prolong life expectancy, enhance a positive lifestyle, as well as many other physiological and psychological benefits.

Isn't it fascinating how many problems you can solve with fitness and exercise! One single practice added to your life can ultimately turn your life around for good! If everyone would just exercise, imagine how many improvements could be experienced in different households, diverse communities, and even countries around the world.

Notably, all these benefits are interrelated to give you a complete state of health and happiness. Therefore, you need to pay close attention to them all by being conscious of each aspect and noting the changes. You may often need to reread some parts of this book at some points for clarity, but remember that this isn't the end of the road. You don't have to limit yourself to what you read here alone; make efforts to watch videos and read other books, too. This will develop your knowledge and ensure you know what you are doing.

Now, it's normal for you to feel overwhelmed or incapable of the journey ahead. You might be thinking, "I don't have the required level of endurance," or, "I've never been committed to something this serious before," or worse, "I can't afford the time, money, and discipline needed for this." At this point, I'd like to remind you what we discussed about making excuses—don't do it. You have a reason and a desire to change your life, that's why you chose to read this book!

We've not come all the way to quit now. You may not have the financial capacity to sign up at the gym, or the discipline to commit to these responsibilities, and you may already be entangled in so many things before now; however, it's the decision you make here now that matters. Keri Russell once said, "Sometimes it's the smallest decisions that can change your life forever."

Your mind can only achieve what you believe. All you need to do is stay focused. Ruminate on it and decide. List all possible obstacles and eliminate them one at a time. Draw your inspiration from successful individuals in this field.

Since you have the knowledge and information needed to initiate a better lifestyle, what will your decision be? Anton Chekhov couldn't have said it better when he stated, "Knowledge is of no value unless you put it into practice."

People strive to get information because actions and decisions can't exist without it. Thus, treasure this information and implement it. You can share it with your partner or friends who desire to walk on this same path. If you've been on this path before now, then it's time for you to increase your pace and frequency, getting better at it. You are still going to learn many things along the way, but the majority of them will be experiences from the uphill and downhill occurrences you encounter.

Furthermore, if you are consistent and dedicated, people will start seeking advice and guidance from *you*. Carry along as many people as you can. Inspire people around you by your actions. Create a sense of purpose for your life, beyond the norms of society. Remember to have fun and make every victory count.

I hope you'll look back one day when you've achieved most of your goals in building a healthy lifestyle and remember the contributions of this book in getting you where you are.

Good luck and Godspeed!

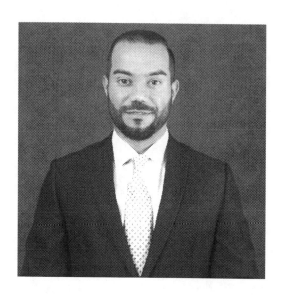

ABOUT THE AUTHOR

With his perspective in life, Sean Yaghotian writes about current conditions of humanity, health, enlightened lifestyle, fitness, and spirituality. Sean concentrates on creating an improved and advanced generation of healthful souls for today's world and tomorrow. His vision is to expand his scholarly concepts and studies across the globe by exploring deep into human anatomy both physically and psychologically, as well as spiritually.

His background and education in corporate communications and entrepreneurship studies derives from the Tier 1 University of Houston, one of the best schools in the U.S. with some of the nation's most prominent and influential leaders and entrepreneurs, such as Houston Mayor Sylvester Turner, Tillman Fertitta, presidential candidate Elizabeth Warren, and the famous NASA astronaut Bruce McCandless II, who was the first to fly untethered in space.

Sean grew up playing basketball, and from a young age had a strong passion for sports, fitness, and bodybuilding. As Sean states, "I've had a long journey with many failures as well as success stories, but the key to my continued growth has been fitness, understanding mindfulness, and my persistence to continue to discover and grow as a human."

Sean is an inventor and United States patent holder. He is a founding member of ZEG Solutions LLC, a MSP technology company in Houston. In addition, he founded A.I. Robotic Technologies, which concentrates on developing innovative technologies focusing on practices that can help individuals with psychological disorders acquire mental clarity, expand their spiritual capacity, and deliver self-healing effects.

Printed in the United States
by Baker & Taylor Publisher Services